FIT FOR THE *FUTURE*

Jeanette Winterson

Jeanette Winterson was born in Lancashire in 1959. After a long tussle with a family of Evangelicals and a short spell at an Ancient University, she moved to London where she still manages to live and work, and lift weights every day. She has written two novels, *Oranges Are Not the Only Fruit* (Pandora, 1985), winner of the 1985 Whitbread Award for First Novel, and *Boating for Beginners* (Methuen, 1985), and edited a selection of short stories on the subject of *Romance*. Spinach is her favourite food.

FIT FOR THE FUTURE

THE GUIDE FOR WOMEN WHO WANT TO LIVE WELL

Jeanette Winterson

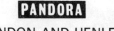
PANDORA

LONDON AND HENLEY

First published in 1986
by Pandora Press (Routledge & Kegan Paul plc)

14 Leicester Square, London WC2H 7PH, England

Broadway House, Newtown Road,
Henley on Thames, Oxon RG9 1EN, England

Set in 9/11pt Palatino
by Columns of Reading
and printed in Great Britain
by the Guernsey Press Co Ltd,
Guernsey, Channel Islands

British Library Cataloguing in Publication Data

Winterson, Jeanette

Fit for the future: the guide for women who want to
live well.—(Pandora handbooks.)
1. Physical fitness for women
I. Title
613.7'045   RA781

ISBN 0-86358 053 X (c)
     0-86358 072 6 (pb)

CONTENTS

For Kate Figes, the best of guinea pigs

CHAPTER 1

BODY POLITIC

Men have broad shoulders and narrow hips and accordingly they possess intelligence. Women have narrow shoulders and broad hips. Women ought to stay at home; the way they were created indicates this, for they have broad hips and a wide fundament to sit upon, keep house and bear and raise children.

Martin Luther, 1531

You owe it to yourself to be beautiful. You should write this phrase on the wall over your bed, in the bathroom, in your diary, on your babies' bib, in your computer programme. Graffiti it in the toilet at work or scratch it on your desk at school. Repeat it in times of stress, shout it in traffic jams. Most important of all believe it. The future is built upon the present which is why you cannot hope for a better time – you can only create one. This book offers no miracles, it demands that you concentrate on yourself and fulfil your own extraordinary potential; there are no solutions that you don't already possess.

Wild beauty is about reaching and maintaining that potential. It's physical freedom, mental sharpness and self respect. Sex and glamour but also confidence and strength. Forget the magazines and the models; you're unique, and any fitness programme you choose, any results you want are up to you, what counts is a lively, irrepressible and highly personal relationship with your own body.

PHYSICAL THINKING

Imagination is the first and foremost stretch exercise. You can't be fit without thinking fit. Whatever state you're in now isn't your pre-ordained lot, you have the power to change, providing you're prepared to look at your body and your life and think beyond them into the state you'd prefer. The body is a place of expression, it reflects the way you live. If you're overweight, overtired, overstressed, exercise alone will alleviate those symptoms but exercise alone can't alter what caused them in the first place. You need a revolution. A fit body will provide the right base and enough energy for change, you have to use your imagination to do the rest. You're beginning a love affair with yourself, so take good care of yourself and decide that from now on, you owe yourself only the best.

FITNESS ROBOTS

Fitness robots are beguiled by size 10, obsessed with weighing eight stone, frantic about their inner thighs and guilty about eating Mars bars. They want to be fit, but to them being fit means whatever the latest fibre diet or media personality exercise programme dictates. They are utterly seduced by the vogue of the moment; it used to be flapper tight chests or eighteen inch waists – now it's a slender androgyny and no stomach. Fitness robots don't think imaginatively about themselves – they adore the fitness package which depends entirely on cause and effect; if you do or buy X then you will achieve Y. Both X and Y are always very specific; a product is offered complete in itself with a predictable end in view. Our society likes packages and while they can sometimes be very useful why tolerate an off the peg mentality when it comes to re-designing your own body? Fitness is fast becoming a major guru to take away the sins of the world (in particular, as with all religions, the sins of womankind) and its message must be simple and seductive. The fitness package doesn't exist to teach you the relationship between mind and body or to understand how to harness your abilities into a creative whole; it exists to isolate the parts so that you can look the part; it's just bend stretch, till you're tired out, then home to wash the leotard. Why settle for being a fitness robot when with a bit of physical thinking you can create yourself in your own image instead of plodding along in someone else's? This book will supply you with the information you need to pursue your own fitness programme in your own way, assuming an initial target time of three months, after which you can measure your progress and adjust accordingly. Think about yourself, think positive and think whole. If your determination is equal to your desire you can have what you want . . . starting now.

CHAPTER 2

BEING THERE

I honestly believe that muscular women are the women of the future. We want strong muscles to match our strong personalities.
Toyah Wilcox, Fitness Magazine, September 1984

Getting fit is a present tense activity. You don't get fit and then stop – there are targets along the way, but no final goal. Being fit becomes a part of you, a condition that exists as long as you do, and changes as you change. At different times in your life you'll want different things from your body; the process you're about to begin never ends and never fixes itself, it's about balance and adjustment and progress. Progress doesn't only mean getting better, progress recognizes change. The way you're fit now won't be the way you're fit in twenty years. That doesn't mean you peak and decline because you get older, it means that your body adjusts perfectly to the changes it undergoes. The important thing is to be equipped to your potential at any stage in your life. This applies to women with disabilities or specific illnesses. Some things can't be overcome, but they can be ameliorated – we have to explore the limits of the possible. This process is an adventure. You will encounter resistance in yourself and from others, you'll want to give up and go back to bed, you'll be frightened and exhilarated by turns and very often you will be surprised. One thing is certain; getting fit will alter your life inevitably and forever. Here's what you need in order to begin:

EQUIPMENT

Buy the best you can afford. Fitness is a present to yourself, so be indulgent. If you buy any clothes that make you look like a small elephant or a sack of vegetables you'll be depressed before you start. Whatever your shape there are sports clothes to flatter it. Go out and find things you want to wear, try the stuff on, bend in it, stretch in it, take no notice of shop assistants who are tanned and size 10. Ask if you want to know anything and don't leave until you're satisfied. Buy colours that suit you, buy something daring and different and make sure you drag along a best friend to bolster you up if you're the doubting type. If you buy a grey tracksuit with a hood and shapeless trousers you are most likely doomed. There is nothing so uninspiring as a grey tracksuit and I have never yet seen anyone look good in one. For some reason they seem to come in only one size and that size will not be your size. You can buy track trousers, T-shirts and sweat shirts separately and this seems to be the best idea because you can then swap and co-ordinate as you like. It seems to be true that the fitter you become and the more you like your body, the less you will want to wear when training. It's a pleasure to see your muscles move, to watch how lithe you are. A pleasure for onlookers, too, so be prepared for the shorts and vest stage or, if you are so inclined, the leotard.

Shoes are very important: you must support your feet and ankles properly depending on what kind of activity you choose. For general purposes, go for NIKES or NU BALANCE or if you feel especially proud of yourself, REEBOKS. You will acquire more than one pair as your interest grows. If you intend to do a lot of stretch and dance, go for a specialist dance shoe. These are light and flexible and they come in pretty colours. At the sports shop of your choice, tell them what you'll be doing, and find out what's on offer. Don't just rush in and snatch the nearest pair of tennis shoes.

I believe in having a completely separate kit for

fitness, including towels and shower accessories and socks. Get a bag, (unless you intend to use a cycle pannier) and stock it with goodies; your favourite shampoo, nail scissors, talc, plasters, toothpaste, spare socks and knickers and small but thick towels. You don't want to carry too much and large towels are cumbersome. Sports towels are designed to be small but effective. They cost more, but they're worth it. You'll need about four unless you're keen on doing the laundry. Body oil is a good thing for after sport because sweating and showering dry out. Get a non greasy sort and use it often, it'll do wonders for your skin tone and add to that healthy glow that will soon become your natural state. If you don't use a perfume or cologne, find one. As your body gets used to continually exfoliating, and your pores stop clogging up you will absorb scents more easily and exude them more potently. There is nothing so delightful as always smelling faintly of a combination of oil and perfume on top of a clean body. Even cats notice it. *Living well and being well is a combination of discipline and self indulgence . . .*

DISCIPLINE

Now you've got the clothes, you need the framework. No one can start getting fit without introducing a new discipline into their lives. It's a discipline that will actually make the rest of your life easier once you get used to it. At first it will be awful. A fundamental part of well-being is to make time for the things you want rather than to let things happen. You should set aside an hour, at least, three times a week for concentrating wholly on your body. It doesn't much matter when that hour is, it doesn't even matter if you shift it around, what matters is that you don't skip it. You will have to take a look at your existing commitments and see what you can move. You're not wasting time, you're learning how to get more out of the time available, and before long your energy levels will have increased so dramatically, that you'll be able to spend extra time in the gym and still achieve as much as you need to elsewhere. This may seem far fetched, but so did building the Eiffel tower or walking on the moon: what seems impossible one day happens the next and there's no reason why it shouldn't happen to you. In true superwoman fashion you'll burst out of a telephone box and re-order your world. So decide now, when you're going to start all this, tell your friends and lovers and don't let anything get in your way.

INDULGENCE

In order to live well you have to be selfish sometimes. You need time for walks, baths, books and entirely self indulgent shopping trips, not the ones where you squash that new frock you wanted in between two toilet rolls and six cans of dog food. You need fresh air, fresh fruit, good sex and a sense of humour. If you don't have a sense of humour try reading *Cold Comfort Farm* (Stella Gibbons) or get out a video of 'Young Frankenstein'. Take time off to look at beautiful things, paintings, sculpture, animals. Above all, don't drink cheap wine unless you're on holiday abroad where the climate will compensate for most things. In England you have to be more careful.

Indulge your body, shower it, sauna it, take it to the sun. If you haven't had enough sensuality in your life, now's the time to make up for it. Champagne and fresh pasta and weekends in bed with your lover or your cat will all give you a healthier attitude towards your body. As you get fitter, you will literally become more alive, you'll feel everything more acutely and you'll start to live through your body in a very direct way. You'll be finding a natural balance and that's best explored by giving way to your fantasies now and again and doing exactly what you like. Women don't know how to indulge. We worry about the washing up or the work we promised to do over the weekend; we try and spend our leisure time productively, which usually means busy doing nothing. So why not do nothing? As you enjoy your body, your mind can relax and after your mind has been able to relax it becomes more alert. Indulgence is just as important as discipline, so don't get all excited about your workouts and forget your long walks, good friends and favourite movies. Do what you like, but do it for pleasure, and don't settle for second best. With a first rate body, why should you?

MIRROR, MIRROR ON THE WALL

I hope you have a full length mirror where you live because you need one. Now that you've decided to make the time, we have to start with the pain. Take off your clothes and take a long hard look at yourself. How do you stand? Is your posture what it should be? How do you distribute your weight? Are your shoulders open or hunched? Does your tummy sag? Do the backs of your arms wobble? Clothes will cover these things, but now you have to be honest with yourself. Poke yourself. Too much flesh? What's your skin like? Do you enjoy what you see? Do you find yourself desirable? Now go and write down exactly what you feel about your body, in detail. Mirror work is vital because we get a chance to quietly examine what we usually don't want to see. You must be absolutely ruthless with yourself about this, no matter how much you hate it, you have to look at your body, in detail, week after week. Soon it will become a pleasure. Move your arms around, watch the way the muscles work, look at the anatomy diagram (pp. 10-11) and locate the major muscle groups. In a while you'll know your body so well that you won't need the mirror, you'll know exactly how you're looking or standing – you'll know whether or not you need to concentrate on certain areas of your body or maintain a general workout. You'll develop an internal mirror which will give you extraordinary grace. For now, rely on props. It's important to treat your body as a unit and take care of all of it, but there are probably areas that need more work than others. Everyone has particular strengths and weaknesses. You may have naturally broad shoulders, which means that they'll develop rather more quickly than the rest of you, or you may have a very floppy tummy, which means endless sit-ups and side bends. It's up to you to decide what you need, and you can only do that by experiment and common-sense. Write down the areas you think need work and spend extra time on them, but don't miss out the rest. In order to achieve total fitness you need overall exercise, and in order to get used to your body, you need to look at it. So, each morning, do just that.

WHAT TO AIM FOR

In a society obsessed with weight and jean size, I hardly need include a height/weight chart, and I'm not going to. You need to use your mirror and your good sense to determine whether or not the weight you are is the weight you want to be. Scales are a very rough guide, the way you look and the way you feel are much more accurate indicators. Muscle is heavier than fat and if you're underweight or comfortably proportioned now, you will probably gain some weight according to the scales as you gain more muscle. At the same time, you could easily drop a size in clothes. What you're going to do is redesign your body according to your own desires and your natural potential. If you're carrying too much fat around you'll start losing it as soon as you start exercising consistently and thinking carefully about what you're eating, when you're eating it and why. The focus for you isn't body weight but body shape, and the only thing that gives your body shape, is muscle. Fat has no shape, it just lies around, so even if you've been scales obsessed and feel that you're the 'right' weight your body might not have much in the way of contour because you've never bothered to tone it, and the little bit of fat you do have will still lie over your frame like an old sheet

9

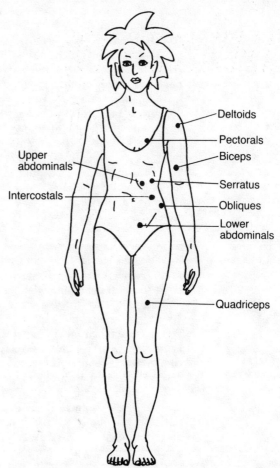

FIGURE 1

with a few bones poking through here and there. Muscle keeps fat controlled and allows you to look nourished and strong out of clothes, as well as OK in them. When you decide what you'd like from your body, there's nothing wrong with a bit of preening; if the idea of visible stomach muscles turns you on then go for it; if you want a very tight bum, then set about creating one. It's often helpful to have a purely self-indulgent fantasy that becomes a

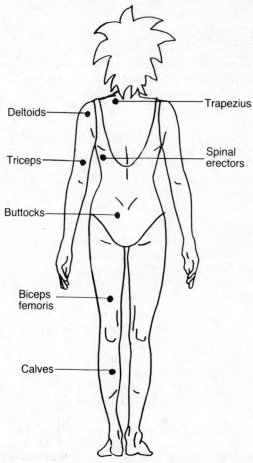

FIGURE 2

reality. It can be the one thing that keeps you going on the days you wish you were a slug again. Picture your body as you would like it to be (remembering that you won't get taller or younger) and make yourself in your own image. You should set an initial target time of three months, then reassess yourself, keeping a record of your progress as you go along. Be realistic but don't aim low, those first three months are going to be hard work!

ACTION

Now you know what you need to start, let's look at the practical ways of changing your body and ultimately your life. What matters is your metabolism. This is the mechanism that converts food into body energy. Everyone has an individual metabolic rate, the rate at which we grow new cells, keep ourselves warm and generally functioning. Exercise speeds up the metabolic rate, not only during activity, but for as long as twenty-four hours afterwards. So, an active woman uses up more energy (calories) while resting than a woman who takes no exercise and, interestingly, more than the woman who takes no exercise and who is also on a diet. This is because our bodies were designed for survival, and so they interpret lack of food as a crisis situation, and begin to conserve energy by slowing down the metabolic rate, so that less energy (calories) is used up. So forget the crash diet.

Exercise promotes weight loss by adjusting our metabolic rate; by using up more energy. If you work out or involve yourself in sport three or four times a week you will enjoy a highly efficient metabolism that converts your food intake properly. No more sluggish feelings and, best of all, the freedom to blow out every now and again on booze or food without having to worry. If you want to start exercising or weight loss you don't need to choose the most demanding activity. It's better to choose something you can do for a longer period, because the forms of exercise which promote the greatest increase in metabolic rate are rhythmic endurance activities, like running, swimming and cycling and in some cases, sex, but you shouldn't imagine you can change your life by bed alone. Use it as an extra. Roughly speaking one pound of fat is worth 4,000 calories, and by looking at the chart you can see what a number of activities cost you in terms of calories. If you're new to exercise and/or overweight, you must include swimming or cycling or both in your programme, for the reasons cited above, and because they work the larger muscle groups (see anatomy diagram) which gives you an all over stretch and tone. Swimming in particular will help you to get over those awful aches and pains that follow your first attempts at vigorous exercise.

If you already worry that you eat too much and some person tells you that exercise will make you want to eat more, ignore them. Exercise raises the blood sugar level; it is when this level drops that we get hungry. Exercise also raises the body temperature which naturally depresses the appetite. Most important, a lot of people suffer from artificial hunger, their appetites don't correspond to their bodily needs, they eat for other reasons or they eat out of habit. With regular exercise the appetite begins to parallel with what we really need, so that we take in as much or as little food as we require for maintenance. Activity is the true state for our bodies, not inactivity. We were built to move and when we stop moving we start functioning artificially, we get out of alignment, both mentally and physically. If you are now unfit and/or overweight, you will be amazed at how different you will be in just a few months. You'll have balance, confidence and instincts you can rely on. You won't be worried about overeating because it will no longer be an issue, and if you've been used to habitual dieting to keep yourself at what you think is an acceptable weight, you'll never have to do it again. You'll be free. Imagine caging tigers, never letting those animals move. No matter how well you fed them, how well you groomed them, they'd be listless. Our bodies are the same, they're incredibly powerful and designed to do extraordinary things. If you sit around, drive around, slop about, of course you'll feel listless, of course you'll eat and drink too much. You're denying yourself a fundamental need. MOVEMENT! So how are you going to start moving? There are two basic choices:

1 at home either alone or with friends
2 at a gym or fitness classes

I am a supporter of gyms and classes for a number of excellent reasons.

1 In the early stages of your physical adventure you'll want to give up and you'll make excuses. If you decide to work out at home, you'll find it much easier to distract yourself with other pseudo-worthy projects, you'll even find cleaning the cat tray exciting. The telephone will ring, the post will arrive, you'll find yourself irresistably drawn to the kitchen for one more cup of tea before you start. If you try and do it at home after work, there'll be the lure of the gin bottle and that programme you have to video. This can be combated if you are strong willed or if you bring in friends, but it seems like adding extra effort to a task that is already hard work. Once you get hooked, you'll want to exercise at home as well, but to start with, especially when the aches set in, you're going to need all the help you can get.

2 You have to prioritize your fitness – don't treat it like a second cousin in the spare room. What you put in is what you get out, so if you have a half-hearted attitude you'll end up with a half-hearted body. Going out to a special place shows commitment. You can't do anything else in a gym except concentrate on your body, not only will this improve your chances it will also clear your mind.

3 Money again. When I tell people what I spend on my club fees, equipment and indulgences, they usually say they could never afford it, though it works out at under £10 a week. When they tell me how much they spend on wrecking their bodies, I point out that being fit is actually going to be cheaper. What you should spend on being fit depends on what you earn and what that earning demands of you. If you have more time than money, then you should look out for the various off-peak schemes and reductions available to anyone without paid work or on a part-time income. There is an increasing number of these schemes and the

standard of instruction is usually very high. If you have more money than time and want to train around your working day, then it's going to be worth shelling out for a gym near your job. You will be able to get there quickly, do what you have to do, and leave showered and refreshed. This is by far the most successful way of training and it quickly becomes a habit. What's more, if you've actually spent the money you're much more likely to go. Most clubs work on a yearly subscription basis with special classes as extra, so to get your money's worth, you'll have to use it. In winter though, you will save on hot water bills.

4   Women don't join clubs in the way that men do – they tend to focus more around the home. This is isolating and dulling. If you join a club you have immediately altered your world to some extent. You will meet new people, get different perspectives and have somewhere to go when life is all too much. Most gyms stay open late. If I feel furious with something or someone, and I can't face a movie or the pub, or if I just want to be by myself, I go to the gym. It's a wonderfully calming and exclusive feeling. You're in control; it's your place, you paid for it, and you can forget the rest of them. It's for these reasons that men are so desperate to hang onto their boys' clubs; the sanctuaries they set up for themselves are denied to women, but now we can make our own. Clubs have excellent facilities for their members, there's more to a gym than the weights room and swimming pool. Shop around, get the best for your money and find somewhere with an atmosphere you like.

5   You'll get the support you need because people concerned with fitness are by and large concerned with other people's fitness too. You'll find people to talk with, people to help you if have a problem with something, and a sense of not doing it alone. Plus there are some beautiful bodies to inspire you.

6   It's difficult to start from scratch without the right props. You can use dumb bells and floor exercises at

home, and you can swim or run or cycle, but you won't have the equipment to tackle the problem area most efficiently. To tone up and build up you need weights, and not many people have the space or the cash to set up their own multi-gym. Of course, you can get fit anywhere if you're determined enough, but I am concerned with time, energy and results. If we want results within our three month experiment, either we work like demons or we use gym facilities.

In order to get the most out of your life and your body you need three things; STRENGTH, STAMINA and FLEXIBILITY. Assuming that I've convinced you to join a gym of some kind, let's consider what these assets involve, and the best ways to increase them using the facilities available.

STRENGTH

Strength is muscle. Healthy muscles are smooth to touch, resilient and springy. They are never slack and they support the internal organs. Look at the anatomy diagram and locate the important muscles:

ABDOMINALS: Usually weak in women. These determine whether the stomach is flat or full.
PECTORALS: These support the breasts and get slacker as we get older.
DORSALS: These are the upper back muscles.
ERECTORS: Lower back.

The others are marked on the diagram, but it is the ones above that we can tone up most quickly. Once your major muscle groups are in good order you'll find it easier to work on fiddly specifics like biceps/triceps, calves/neck etc. Women tend to have naturally strong legs; you should be able to build and firm your legs quite easily as you go along. Arms will be more of a problem and may need extra work unless you carry things a lot.

Muscle strength is literally what keeps you upright. If your back muscles are weak you will tend to slump, your shoulders will round, and if you have to sit or stand for long periods you will develop aches and pains, particularly in the lower back. Muscle strength also protects your joints; the stronger you are, the less likely you are to injure your joints, and if you do, strong muscles will compensate for the damage. So much for that, but you know and I know that muscle tone looks good. At the moment you might not see much muscle as you stand in front of your mirror, but soon your body will gain definition, not bulging biceps but a measured and obvious line. How? WEIGHTS!

Weight training is the most wonderful thing in the world. There is nothing to compare with the mental and physical exhilaration of watching your body in action. You have to use weights in front of a mirror to make sure you keep your body properly aligned. It's entirely narcissistic and the better you get the more pleasurable it is. When you first decide to use weights it's better to have instruction than to try and do it out of any book. An instructor will decide what weights you should be using, what your targets ought to be and show you how to lift and balance. For women, most of whom are not concerned with becoming beefcakes, weights are a comprehensive and imaginative way of finding our bodies' potential and learning how to be graceful. Animals are graceful because they know instinctively how to carry and control their body mass, most of us who are not dancers, athletes or lucky, don't have such instincts. Weights will retrain you. You will come to understand how your muscles work in isolation and together. You will have to focus on your body in quite a different way. For a while it will be like watching a stranger and then you will realize you are becoming a new person. What I'm talking about here are free weights, dumb-bells and bar bells. There are two other valuable options: Multi-gym and Nautilus equipment.

MULTI-GYM

This is exactly what it sounds like. A fixed piece of machinery with a number of different functions. You

17

move around it using the different bits. You don't need much instruction to use one of these because it's designed to make it quite difficult to hurt yourself, and there are no free weights to drop on your foot or find yourself stuck underneath. The important thing, as in all exercise, is to keep your body aligned. If you twist or pull at an angle to the equipment you're using, then you'll get hurt. You need to be smooth, rhythmic and controlled. If you've never done any weights before and the gym you choose has a multi-gym and free weights, start on the multi-gym and stay with it for about a month. After a month you'll have more confidence and you'll be noticing an improvement, then you can add free weights to your programme, which are certainly more absorbing and less boring. Multi-gyms do the job, but they're inflexible; there isn't much room for experiment. You might, of course, decide you adore them, in which case stick with it!

NAUTILUS

There is a Nautilus machine for every muscle group in the body. The machines work by isolating a particular muscle group and allowing you to work on it while leaving the rest of your body in a state of relaxation. They're space age machines that will tone, trim and build your body faster than anything else you can do. If you have limited time, you can do a full Nautilus workout in around half an hour. Follow that with something aerobic like swimming or cycling (fixed cycles will do) and you've done the best by your body. What's more, you've done the whole of your body. A typical Nautilus workout involves twelve to fifteen machines. The amount of weight you shift is selected according to your strength, but the aim is to make it so heavy that you can't move it more than ten times – if you can do more than twelve you need a heavier weight. Nautilus is a great shape improver and if you want quick results, this is the equipment you should be going for. All Nautilus gyms come with instructors who will design a programme specially for you. Not surprisingly, these gyms are usually more expensive than ordinary weights/multi-gym, mainly because each piece of Nautilus costs over £2000. We're talking about the Porsche end of the market, but with enormous advantages that seem to me to make the extra outlay worth it. Nautilus is valuable at whatever stage or age you are. I use it as the basis of my workout, followed by free weights, and since I'm always pushed for time, it's comforting to know that I can keep myself in shape that way. Once you reach a certain level, maintenance gets easier. I always do one long workout a week, no matter what else is happening, but a couple of other days just on the Nautilus or in the pool will be enough – enough to stay as I am; if I wanted to push further, I'd have to work harder again. There are special Nautilus machines and programmes for pregnant women, that concentrate on improving back, thighs and upper body, the areas which are having to carry the extra weight. Women seem to want to use Nautilus more than men do, mainly because it doesn't have the associations that come with lifting weights. (Positive for men, negative for women.) This is wrong thinking, but if it gets women onto the machines, it has some use. Once your body starts to improve, you'll want to explore other ways of continuing the process and, after all, when you can lift weights gracefully, (which most men can't) it doesn't look butch and it does approach an art form. If you don't believe me, go and watch a woman who can do it.

If you can afford it, (and you probably can if you really want to) joint a Nautilus gym. Most of them offer a free trial workout so that you can see what you're in for, and most will take time and trouble over your individual requirements. If you don't know anything about training and/or you're pushed for time, this is the equipment for you.

Weight training isn't the only way of improving muscle strength, but it is the simplest, because to gain strength you have to work your muscles against a load which can be either your own body or a weight. If you want to gain strength you have to keep increasing the amount of work you do, it's no good simply repeating the same exercises for the same time every day, you must either increase the weight, or the speed at which you perform a particular exercise or the number of repetitions of an exercise. It's actually a mistake to use weights every day because your body needs time to settle down and deal with what you're doing to it. Three times a week for one hour is ideal and if you find you want to train more often, then do something else, like swimming or a dance class or some kind of competitive sport. Remember to do your warm ups before you start – if you miss them your body will have to work harder for no reason and no benefit. All that will happen is that you will get tired more quickly and ache more totally afterwards. Warm ups give your body the warning it needs to get ready for strenuous exercise. Stiffness and soreness occur the day after a workout and may last for two days. It always hits hardest those who have just started because the muscles aren't firm enough to cope with the extra workload. The only way to alleviate stiffness is to keep exercising! No matter how bad you feel, (providing you're not injured) don't let more than two days elapse between workouts. If you do, especially to start with, you'll keep hitting the same problems and your progress will be very much slowed down. Resign yourself to pain and get that part over with as quickly as possible by sticking to your discipline. If you do find that part of your body is so sore that you can't use the weights (fixed or free) exercise that part thoroughly and gently with your warm ups and spend the rest of the time on other, less painful areas. The important thing is to keep moving once you've started. Water exercises and swimming are both good ways of looking after a sore body.

STAMINA

Stamina is really your heart and lung rating and this is where aerobics comes in. Aerobic fitness is your bodies' ability to work at near maximum pitch over a length of time. If you have stamina you won't fall into a crumpled heap when you run for the bus, nor will you cut a swathe in the pool for all of one lap, then clutch the side for support. Stamina means more staying power and less embarrassment. There are plenty of good looking bodies around, (good looking in clothes!) but the important thing is that those bodies should also be functional. As women we're too often encouraged to be only decorative. The tyranny of diet and fashion dictates a certain desirable shape and size but still says very little about what goes on underneath. I don't see the point of desperately reducing your weight and scrubbing your cellulite to fit into a beach bikini if you don't have the strength and stamina to enjoy the water. Enjoyment is the best thing about being fit; more things are possible and their pleasure factor is greatly enhanced. What actually happens to your body is that your heart beats more strongly and pumps more blood with each stroke. Eventually your heart is able to achieve the same results with less work, and as the muscles in your chest wall get stronger, you'll be able to breathe more easily, and get out of breath less quickly. The best way to increase your stamina is through vigorous exercise which must last at least twenty minutes. Do this by running, swimming, on an exercise bike or at an aerobics class, and fit it in around your weights workout, though at first you probably won't be able to do them in conjunction with each other. Whichever form you choose, remember not to slacken the pace – you have to keep your heart rate up to gain any benefit. I like to swim after weights – you may find you like to cycle first or sign up for a totally separate class. It's up to you, as long as you do it regularly. We'll be looking at specified activities later in the book and deciding what their separate and comparative values are.

FLEXIBILITY

This is the ability to move all your major joints and muscles as nature intended. Children have a suppleness that tends to get lost as they grow up, but this need not be the case; if you put your body (and theirs) through its full range of movement each day you will be protected from injury, stiffness, aches and possibly even arthritic complaints later in life. Whilst you need not train aerobically or with weights more than three times a week, stretching to stay supple is best as a daily activity. It doesn't take long – on the days you're not incorporating your stretches into your training programme, you'll need around fifteen minutes to set your body in motion. I prefer the mornings because it's a positive start to the day. You'll feel better and have the advantage on your sluggish colleagues if you have to go to work. If you're at home, or doing other things, you'll still feel the enormous surge of energy a short stretch can give, and you can use that energy to buoy you up through the day. As your flexibility improves you'll find your other forms of exercise get easier, and you'll learn more poise and grace than any deportment class could offer you. Your flexibility varies according to the time of day – in the morning you'll be stiffer, so make sure to wake yourself up gently with some easy bends and twists before you try and turn yourself inside out. Don't be discouraged if you find something impossible to do in the mornings; practice that movement later in the day, and gradually work towards managing it first thing. Your body will respond, but especially if you're new to exercise, it'll be a bit of a shock for it, so use some of the starters I've suggested below, and then use your own sense and imagination to design a set that suits you. Fitness is creative – once you've got the basics you can build your own patterns . . .

WARM UPS

Warm ups are NOT optional. Without a good overall stretch and get-ready your body won't do what you ask it to in terms of strenuous exercise, without your hurting or straining yourself. You can't walk out of the office and into a gym and expect your body to be ready to perform. Nor can you come home tired and emotional after fighting with life, the universe and everything and expect to work out efficiently without first loosening up. Obviously if you get out of bed and belt down to your gym on a bike, you've already had a good aerobic start. Use your own good sense about your body; if it stays still after you've warmed up, do a bit more. Part of your fitness process is learning to listen to what your body is saying. Soon you'll be able to tell exactly what you need and when you need it, but until then, it's better to play safe and follow a specific routine. The suggestions below are by no means the only way of warming up and stretching out, but they are comprehensive and should provide the right amount of challenge. If you prefer to ignore these and find another system, that's fine.

First of all, BREATHE! Most of us breathe as if air was in short supply. Stand up straight, feet apart, hands on hips, head up and tilted back slightly. Draw in a deep breath through your nose and feel that breath going right up your trunk and into your shoulders. Now exhale slowly through the mouth. Do this until you feel comfortable with it and until you feel your diaphragm has expanded. It's a very straightforward feeling, so don't look for mystery. By and by your breathing will become more efficient and more beneficial, but in the early stages of exercise, it's important that you concentrate on it. If you feel a sudden twinge or pain as you work out, sit or stand with your spine straight and do some deep breathing. This will assist the siezed muscle and alleviate cramps, (though if you've really done yourself in, it won't do much at all). Oxygen is the body's most basic nourishment; don't stint yourself. When you've stopped your deep breathing, continue to breathe fully and regularly and slowly revolve your neck round its circuit. Your chin should drop right forward onto your chest and you should feel a pull at each side of your neck as you move it round. Do this about ten times. Now take your hands from your hips and raise them right above your head as though you were trying to reach something just too high. Point your fingers, throw back your head and go onto tiptoe. Feel the stretch all the way through. Now make your hands into fists and bring both arms down and out at the sides in a crucifixion pose. With your fists still clenched begin a windmill movement swinging the arms with great vigour while keeping them absolutely straight (see diagram). You should build up the number of these you can do both backwards and forwards because it's a wonderful shoulder exercise and very good for releasing tension. Do at least ten each way and try more each time, even if it's only one more.

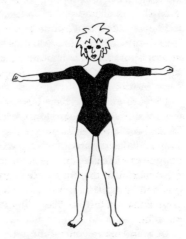

FIGURE 3

Drop your arms back by your side again and prepare for side bends. You should be able to bend sideways so that your fingertips come just below your knee. You'll feel the stretch on your opposite side. This is great for toning the intercostal muscles which are often weak in women. Do ten each side.

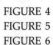

FIGURE 4
FIGURE 5
FIGURE 6

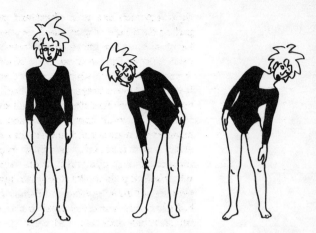

Now put your hands above your head again and bending first to the side sweep right down in a touch-toe movement then come back up the other side until your hands are again above your head. This will call on your stomach and lower back muscles, is quite easy to do and should help your spinal flexibility if you do it properly and regularly. Now for the legs.

Drop down into a racing position, as though you were waiting for the gun to go off for the 200 metres. Make sure your back is straight and that you are balanced. Using the front leg as a support, gently bounce the back leg so that you can feel a pull at the front muscle at the top of the thigh. Keep the stretch position as tight as you can bear it and don't bend your knee on the back leg. Do thirty of these with each leg.

Now lie flat on your back with your hands under your bum and draw up your legs into your chest. Now push your legs straight out, keeping them off the floor and pointing your toes (see diagram). Do as many as you can, always making sure that you bring your legs back up as close to your chest as possible and that you are stretching them out as far as possible. No wobbles or bent knees allowed. This is

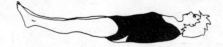

FIGURE 7

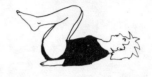

FIGURE 8

good for your thighs and stomach and hip joints, and it supports your back. If you ever hurt your back while doing something or other and find it too painful to do sit ups, then increase the number you do of this exercise, but remember to keep your hands well under your bum (palms down).

The moment had to come when I would mention sit ups, and now that I have let's deal with them. They're painful and horrid and nasty and essential. No matter how fit you become, no matter how wall-like your stomach, sit ups will always make you gasp because they're the sort of thing you just end up doing more of, the fitter you get. If I push myself to do 100, which I do most days, I'm in pain after about 80, so it's not without compassion that I force these things on you. Women often have lousy stomach muscles and mostly they wish they hadn't. The only way to change yours is to start now with as many sit ups as you can do easily, and a few more after that point. You have to push yourself. I do my sit ups on a slanted board because that makes it harder, and if you're at a gym that has a rack, then start low and work up as you want more results. There's nothing wrong with doing them on the floor as long as you hook your feet under something solid so that you don't cheat or slide about. Keep your knees bent and put your hands behind your head. Each time you sit up, breathe out hard and breathe in as you go back. This will help you to avoid strain and give your muscles the extra oxygen they need. If you're really feeble, then do sit ups twice a day, just a few each time. You'll soon tone up, though remember you need to work on the intercostals as well as the abdominals, so don't skimp on those side bends. Later on, I'll offer a few suggestions for extra work on specific areas, for all of you who have a dream. All of these exercises can be used for general flexibility as well as being excellent pre-weights preparation, but if you want real flexibility, you need more. For the stretching exercises listed below, hold the stretch at a point where you feel a comfortable pulling along the extended muscle. Hold this for about fifteen seconds, and do each exercise five times.

HAMSTRINGS AND LOWER BACK

Sit with one leg straight out in frong and the other tucked at 90° with your foot alongside your bum. Sit with your back absolutely straight and breathe as we have already discussed. When you feel comfortable and relaxed in this position, lean forward from your hips over the straight leg reaching for your foot and at the same time getting your head as close to your knee as you can. Eventually you'll get your nose on the floor, but until that happy moment, concentrate on the point at which you feel strain but not pain. Repeat with other leg.

FIGURE 9

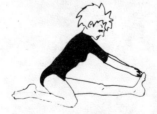

QUADRICEPS

Lie on your stomach and clasp your ankles with your hands. Push in with your heels towards your bum. Remember to keep your head up and don't rock your body.

FIGURE 10

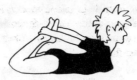

CALVES

Stand up straight, feet together. Go onto tiptoe and lower yourself again, stretching the calf muscle as much as you can. Do this about twenty times and follow it by leaning forwards against a wall (see diagram) and moving your legs backwards as far as you can while keeping your heels on the ground.

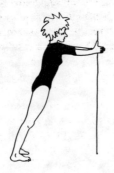

FIGURE 11

KNEE BENDS

Stand with your hands on your hips, bend your knees to make a right angle, then straighten up, keeping your knees straight.

FIGURE 12

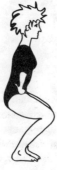

INNER THIGHS

Sit with your legs straight out in front and as far apart as possible. Lean forwards from the hips, keeping your back straight. One day your nose will touch the floor.

FIGURE 13

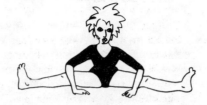

HIP AND BUM

Stand holding something with both hands at about hip height. Without turning your hips raise your right leg out to the side as high as you can, then lower it again. Do about ten with each leg.

FIGURE 14
FIGURE 15

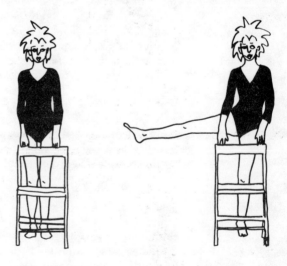

HIPS AND PELVIS

If we were all belly dancers life would be easier, at least as far as flexibility is concerned. Pretend you are. Plant your feet a little apart, put your hands on your hips and make the fullest circles you can with your hips, if you feel like hoolah hooping do so.

29

Then move your hips back and forth and sideways, try writing letters with your body. It's fun, and you'll get more and more inventive about what shapes you can make. It will make your hips much more mobile, cut down on lower back ache, and strengthen your pelvic floor, which amongst other things means better sex because the muscles are tighter without being stiffer. If you leap out of bed late one morning and have time for nothing more, do a bit of belly dancing in the bathroom as you clean your teeth. Belly dance as you make the toast, gyrate as you grind the coffee, it may feel a little strange at first, but it's good for you!

THOSE PROBLEM AREAS

Genetics play a large part in how you'll be able to develop your body. Some areas will come on faster than others, and some will take a great deal of effort for only average results. No one can tell you in advance how your body will respond. I, for instance, have to spend 50 per cent more time on my legs just to keep them in proportion to my shoulders and back which build muscle very easily. Some women have strong legs and weak calves, some will have to work for hours on their arms. Just don't worry. Keep yourself in proportion and adjust what exercises you do as you discover more about your body structure. What you mustn't do is to confuse genetics with laziness. You'll have to work hard at first, especially if you've been relying on clothes and the right lighting to cover up some sag.

TUMMIES

You may find, even if you're a suitable weight, that you don't have much in the way of muscle round the middle. If so, do extra work on your abdomen and intercostals. After you've warmed up, do a set of sit-ups, as many as you can, then follow these with side bends. One of the best ways of firming the intercostals is to take a pole, a broom handle will do, lay it across your shoulders, arms stretched along it, and kneeling down turn your trunk from side to side as far as you can go (see diagram). Do around fifty

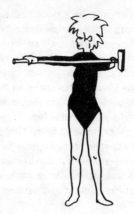

FIGURE 16

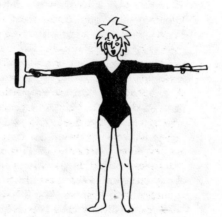

FIGURE 17

of these, keeping your spine straight. Finish your workout in the same way, though if you're using Nautilus you won't need the pole because there is an excellent machine to tone the intercostals. Sit-ups, though are now a feature of the rest of your life; no matter what equipment you use, no matter what sport you do, there's nothing so good as sit-ups. Flat on the floor is fine, but a slant board is better. Eventually you can hold a weight behind your head too, just to increase the agony.

Don't forget that the leg-in exercise I told you
about in the warm-up section is superb for keeping
the flab away from the lower abdomen. Because
muscles don't work independently, but in conjunction with each other, it's also necessary to exercise
the lower back if you want to keep your waist in
shape. One of the best ways to do this, to increase
strength and reduce stiffness, are back bends: stand
with feet apart, hands on hips. Bend straight
backwards at the waist as far as you can without
losing your balance, then pull yourself upright using
your stomach muscles only. Now bend backwards at
an angle to the right and pull yourself up, then at an
angle to the left. This may be a strain at first, so
don't do too many, but do build up the number of
repetitions as you are able.

FIGURE 18
FIGURE 19
FIGURE 20

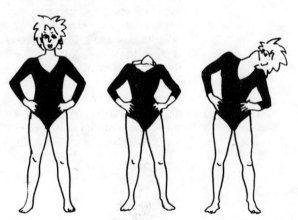

BUMS

A tight bum is fun. Here's how to get one.

Rear leg raises

Lie on your stomach, upper body raised and
supported on your elbows. Raise your right leg up
behind you as far as you can, without much knee
bending, then lower it slowly to the floor again.
Repeat with other leg. Start with five, then ten then
fifteen each leg.

Leg lifts

Hold onto something at about hip height; without turning your hip raise one of your legs out to the side as far as it'll go, then lower it. Do the same with the other leg.

Lunges

Good for upper legs and hips too. Stand with your feet together, arms out at the sides for balance. Step forward with your right leg and sink on it till the knee of your left leg touches the floor. Stand up straight again and do the exercise with the other leg. When your muscles start to shake, stop! This exercise is a wonderful balance and flexibility improver.

BOSOMS

If you must improve your bust you'll have to build your pectoral muscles, because they're the ones that hold you up. To really work these muscles you need equipment; again, Nautilus is very good, because it actually has a machine for women's chests. Dumbbells and push ups, though, will work just as well, though they will take longer. Don't be afraid of push-ups, they're hard for women at first, and you'll feel silly when you fall over with your nose in the dirt, but they're worth the effort; build up the amount you can do until you reach fifteen or twenty – that will keep you toned. Push-ups work mostly

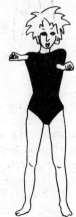

FIGURE 21

on the centre of the pectorals, try this for toning the outsides of the muscle: stand with your feet apart, arms held out at the side, slowly cross your arms, then return them to their first position. Repeat, this time crossing left over right, or the opposite of what you've just done (see diagram).

If you're using weights, take a pair of dumb bells that are a comfortable strain, lay flat on your back, arms out at the sides holding the dumb bells, then slowly raise your arms simultaneously until they're straight out in front of you, pointing at the ceiling. Lower regularly, don't let gravity whizz your arms to the floor. Do as many as you can, until the muscle starts to shake.

TRICEPS

If ever a woman had an under-used muscle, it's this one. Even if you tone your shoulders and biceps, you'll have saggy arms unless you work on this muscle at the back (it lies behind the bicep and as the name suggests is composed of three elements or heads, all of which need to be taken into consideration). If you're not sure about your triceps, hold up your arm and see if you can wobble it about three inches down from the armpit. Chances are you can;

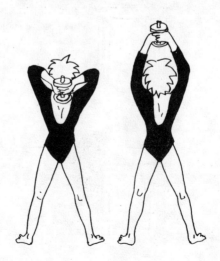

FIGURE 22
FIGURE 23

here's how to firm it up. Take a dumb bell, weight according to what feels right to you. Stand with your feet apart and hold the weight behind your neck, so that your elbows stick out at the sides (it's best to do this in front of a mirror) then raise your arms up behind your head, until your arms are straight (see diagram). Lower and repeat. You should do three sets of eight, interchanging them with the following: Stand feet apart, back straight but leaning slightly forward, holding your dumb-bells at ease by your side. Slowly move your arms backwards and outwards, extending them as fully as you can, without feeling any pain across your back. Bring them back by your side and repeat for three sets of eight. Again it's best to check your posture in a mirror because this exercise can easily pull you out of alignment. If you haven't got any weights, arrange two pieces of

FIGURE 24

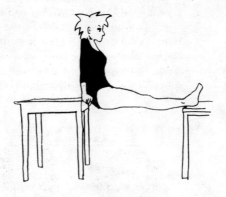

FIGURE 25

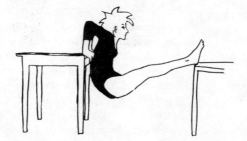

furniture in such a way as to get your feet propped up on one and your upper body balanced on your arms, propped up on another. Now dip your body up and down so that the triceps take the strain (see diagram). Don't be too enthusiastic to start with or you'll literally fall between two stools. This is a very good stretcher and firmer.

A WORD ABOUT BICEPS

Because I have a vendetta against flabby arms, I would encourage you to work separately on your biceps as well as your triceps, no matter what exercise programme you decide to take up. It doesn't take that much extra time, and the results are well worth it. For your biceps, use dumb-bell curls in a series of three movements. Curls will also strengthen your forearms and wrists. Do these in front of a mirror. Stand feet apart, back straight, weights held palm up in front of your thighs. Now raise your arms through 90° until you have a right angle at your elbow joint. Lower and repeat seven times. On the eighth time hold the curl at the right angle and intead of lowering pull up into your chest, then drop back to the right angle. Repeat seven times, then lower to thigh level. For the last seven movements, curl your arms all the way up and back again from thighs to chest, thus incorporating the previous two movements. When you have completed this exercise you will have made twenty-one repetitions. (3×7: remember to keep your elbows in and to breathe steadily.)

Obviously there are many other kinds of exercises that you can do for all of the areas we've discussed. My purpose is to keep this book simple and to encourage you to find them out for yourself. If you are joining a gym, and I hope that you are, make the best possible use of the instructors. Don't be afraid to keep asking, and tell them if anything worries you (if you feel you're working hard for little return, for instance). Alternatively, there are hundreds of exercise books on the market which you should use if you're interested, but as far as I'm concerned,

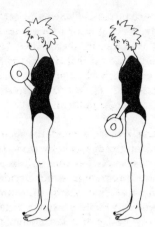

FIGURE 26
FIGURE 27

personal instruction is always the best option. Would you expect to learn the piano via a how-to manual? Learning about your own body has to be a matter of trial and error, common-sense and acts of faith. You have to believe you can change, you have to believe you can develop. I could stuff this book full of exercises which would be of no use at all if you weren't galvanized into using them. I want to convince you that fitness is worth it, and offer a few pointers to get you started; after that this becomes a reference book only, because you'll be getting on with your own adventure and I can't predict what that will be. Remember that every exercise programme is unique to the individual; once you understand what you need to do don't get tied down into an unchanging ritual – alter and develop what you do according to what your body asks of you and what you require from it.

JUNGLE GYM   The law of the jungle operates most fully in the gym, unless you join one with a high proportion of women members. This shouldn't put you off, but you should be aware of it; when you are, it's quite funny. . . . They are Tarzan, you are Jane; at least that's what they'd like to believe. They go along and flex their biceps and sweat and then you come along and flex your biceps and sweat and it upsets them. The first sign of their disquiet is when they start to eye you up; it's not a pick-up, far from it, they're too busy picking up their weights – they want to tell you how to exercise so that they can be sure you're not going to do anything they don't know about. Like doctors, they'll talk about your body as if they understand it better than you do. They'll tell you what you need. I am no longer polite to Tarzans, I no longer say thank you for advice I didn't ask for and can't use, I tell them to go away. This provokes two responses; either a hurt sniff and a warning that I don't know what I'm doing, or a bit of abuse because I'm so ungrateful and they were only trying to help. Either ignore them or lose your temper, don't bother to discuss it because they won't listen. They're upset because you're trampling on their balls. If another woman is teaching you how to use equipment, their interest becomes especially acute; some butt in while others find the urge to stand over you irresistible. They look impatient and indulgent until you've finished with a particular piece of equipment then they leap to use it, increasing the weight as dramatically as possible so that you can see how strong they are and how feeble you are. Not all boys in gyms act like this, some are too busy and some are just well behaved adults, but there'll always be a few who have to be Tarzan and can't help feeling threatened when Jane drops the tea-pot and reaches for the dumb-bell.

The other point to note is that if any piece of equipment seems to you to have been geared for men with no alternative for women's use (some multi-gym apparatus can be fixed too high up, for instance), then complain. You don't have to feel worried about not being at least 5' 8". Similarly, if you can't find the correct weights, because they're all too heavy, make a fuss about it. The YMCA clubs, whilst being excellent and good value sports centres, tend to think in terms of men, not women, when it comes to buying and fixing apparatus. The one in London has a pull-up bar that I have to stand on a stool to reach which is extremely annoying, especially since they have a high percentage of women members. I ought to say that one Tarzan did offer to lift me up . . .

When you choose a gym or sports club, look around it first and try to test some of the machines or weights you'll want to use. Make sure you feel comfortable with the changing and showering facilities and find out what percentage of women use the place. If you're paying for your sport, make sure you're not paying for something that is only partially useful and, if possible, go for somewhere with a few women instructors. There are a number of women's weight training courses on offer and I would advise you to book in for one, if free weights appeal to you. Not only will this keep you out of danger because you can hurt yourself easily, it will also give you the confidence to walk into a weightroom full of Tarzans and not worry about how obsessed with muscle power they are. They believe that you are either envious or full of admiration as they heave about; what they can't believe is that you don't give a damn and are too busy shaping your own beautiful lines. If you handle your own weights skilfully they can't bother you; if they think you're a beginner, they'll be swarming around like overblown wasps. Body builders haven't heard of the Equal Opportunities Commission, all they hear is the call of the wild. This isn't your ball game; what's important is you, your body and what you want to do with it.

WHEN SHOULD YOU EXERCISE?

There are some exercise persons who are more interested in discipline than in self-indulgence. This seems to me to be a highly unbalanced approach and can only lead to public-school type misery. As long as you have determined to spend one hour three times a week on your body (to start with, hopefully you'll enjoy yourself so much you'll do more), that hour doesn't have to be always between 1pm and 2pm or between 6pm and 7pm. Only you can decide the demands of a day and how best to organize it. There's no reson to satellite around fixed points unless such a method is genuinely useful. Especially useless is the mentality that decrees you should spring out of bed very early and beat your body into shape before the milkman delivers. Sleeping doesn't just affect the brain; muscles relax, the circulatory system is naturally very different when you're horizontal rather than vertical, and you need to restore the blood volume level when you get up and before you start moving around. (Blood volume level falls during the night because the kidneys excrete urine, which is why you always want to pee when you wake up, even though you did so before you went to bed and even though you clearly haven't had anything to drink while you've been asleep.) The best way to treat your body when you wake up is to have a peaceful half hour and a large glass of mineral water before you think of doing anything. If you're new to fitness, don't even try to do your workouts before you've been moving around for a few hours, otherwise you'll feel stiff, tired and depressed because your performance seems so inadequate. Gentle stretch exercises are a pleasant and easy way to get yourself perked up, and an early swim can only do you good, but I wouldn't recommend running or weight training or any activity that calls on the whole body to be vigorous rather suddenly. Other times to avoid are after meals – you need a two hour gap, and possibly more if you've been stuffing. If you're sick, don't train, your body needs all its resources to repair the damage. If you train last thing at night, you'll probably stay awake longer than you should because you've just spurred yourself into activity when you're usually soothing yourself into sleep!

THE ECCENTRIC'S GUIDE TO EXERCISE

We've already decided that there isn't enough time in the world to conquer it and enjoy it and do your exercises – at least there isn't if you're going to be unimaginative. Imagination is the first and foremost stretch exercise. You can improve your body almost anywhere at anytime, all you need is a little panache. We've discussed belly dancing, and certainly that's one thing you shouldn't miss out on; if you have your own office or sympathetic colleagues there's no reason why you can't belly dance round the office as well as in the comfort of your own home. The other place to belly dance is the shower, especially if you have a mobile attachment. Take hold of the shower head and ask it to dance then sweep around while you get clean. That way you can strengthen your pelvis and thighs at the same time as exfoliating your gorgeous body with a bath mitt. The other great thing about showers (assuming they have a forceful jet) is that they can be used for massage, the back of the neck being particularly responsive. Stand under the flow so that it hits you directly in the centre of your neck just where it joins the shoulders, then move your head round in a full circle, dropping it right down onto your chest and right back so that the water gushes over your face (remember to keep your mouth closed). This will relax and strengthen your neck, and refresh your facial tissues. If you have a lower back ache, a stronger shower jet coupled with a hoolah hoop movement will cure it far more effectively than a soak in the tub. Put the shower head close to the ache, make sure it's at full strength and as it plays over the injured part make a full circle with your hips, making sure that you can feel the movement in your back. This will free the muscle while the hot water spray relaxes it. Sex in the shower is an excellent all over body toner whether you do it by yourself or with a partner.

There are lots of things you can do in the bath, one of the easiest being leg-raises. Lie back and slowly raise your legs each in turn, say to the level of the top of the tap. Hold for a count of five then lower the leg back into the water. When you get tired of that one, make full circles with your ankles. Ankle exercises always seem to me to be the most tedious, and I tend to skip them in my workout, but I can't find any excuse to skip them in the bath and somehow they don't seem such an imposition. If your bath has handles at the sides you can exercise your triceps wonderfully by doing a version of the dipping exercise mentioned earlier. Raise your upper body on your arms until your arms are locked and fully stretched out (make sure the bath handles aren't slippy) then dip your body back down until your arms return to their original position. Be inventive, design your own exercises for your own bathroom, it may seem a little strange at first, but no stranger than lying in a pool of water in the first place. If you find yourself in a queue out of doors, take the opportunity to do some deep breathing. This will help you keep calm, if that's possible in a queue, and it will give your body a chance to stretch itself on the inside. Concentrate on something pleasing while you breathe, either around you or in your head and think about the air opening you up and feeding your muscles (muscles need oxygen). If you find yourself queueing indoors and the air is such that breathing is a risk anyway, you can console yourself by strengthening your bum and stomach. All you have to do is tighten both as much as possible, then hold for a count of five, then release for a count of five. Keep on doing this until you have made both as tight as possible, or until you have reached the front of the queue. No one will notice and you'll feel better. If you're sitting at a desk and beginning to feel lousy, there are a number of things you can do apart from leaving right away. For tired or cramped legs, stretch each leg out in turn in front of you and hold for a few seconds, you might like to make circles with your feet at the same time. If your shoulders are drooping and aching, sit with your back straight up and pull both shoulders back at the same time, as though you're trying to make them touch. Then bounce them up and down as though you wanted to wrap them round your ears. If you feel really bad, ignore your colleagues, stand up and do some deep knee bends, breathing fully as you move. Suppose you have to go and make a telephone call standing up; this is a superb opportunity to develop your calves, because you can stand on tiptoe then back to flat again without the person on the other end having any idea what you're up to. Of course, if you're in a busy public place, strangers might stare, but then they are only strangers so what does it matter? You could probably fit in about fifty calf stretchers on an average telephone call, and that means fifty you won't have to do in the gym later.

If you're carrying shopping, divide your load as equally as you can and use the two bags as dumb-bells. You can lift them as curls, or you can lift them straight up as shoulder toners and all while you're walking home or standing at the bus stop. Alternatively, if you do a weekly shop that isn't too heavy and you live close enough to home, why not pile it all in a rucksack and run home at a leisurely pace? The brave steely heroes do it all the time, except they wear khaki suits and carry rocks; that's a waste of time, but fetching back the shopping is productive and can be made into a useful exercise as well.

When you go for a walk, be conscious of how you walk. Make sure your shoulders are back, your head is raised, and take steps that stretch your legs as well as simply move you along. Walking is one of the best things you can do, it's the body's fundamental and natural exercise, so make the most of it. Most people could correct their bad posture by thinking about the way they walk. Once you learn to walk easily, powerfully and economically, you're toning your body with every step you take, literally. Sometimes when you walk, try clenching your bum as you go along, it won't show and it won't impede your progress, but it will do wonders for your long-term rear view. Chewing may not seem to you to be much of an exercise, but it can be if you do it with vigour. Our facial muscles don't get a great deal of movement in the average run of things; we frown and smile, but not much else, and the face is full of tiny muscles that would like to move. When you chew, therefore, make the most of your mouth. Other places to involve your face muscles are whilst sitting on the toilet and whilst working at the typewriter. Just screw your face into as many contortions as possible. Soon you'll do it without even noticing, but you will notice the benefits.

IDLING YOUR WAY TO A BETTER BODY

It's not all blood sweat and tears – some of it is glorious self indulgence. You must take time to appreciate yourself, and this is best done generally lying around being peaceful and feeling good. Every woman needs inertia in her life because most women are twice as busy as most men, juggling with jobs and homes and children and dogs and thousands of other tasks that the boys ignore. Even if you can only manage it at weekends, or for just half an hour after your workout you should find a warm or sunny place, make yourself comfortable and relax body and mind. I don't even suggest that you read or listen to music. Above all don't knit. Allow yourself a space that is simply for you and think about what a wonderful person you are and how lucky all your friends are to know you, how privileged your lover is to be able to take you to bed, how blessed are your animals that you are their protector. It doesn't matter if you indulge in hyperbole, you probably underestimate yourself most of the time, so a little redress can only do you good. Think about your body and how you've begun to improve and enjoy it. Feel it, feel the new muscle and the firmer curves, it's yours and you should be proud of yourself.

Now and again give yourself an early night, if

possible without a lover around. Usually we go to sleep dog tired and quite late, with a head full of tomorrow's demands and today's complications. You deserve a light supper, some fine wine and a few free hours under the duvet. This is one of the most regenerating things you can do. It will totally relax you and clear you out for a fresh start. If you find that you sleep for hours and still wake up tired, you need a break, a proper one for a few days; that's a clear message from your body and you can't ignore it unless you want to get sick. One of the troubling things about taking your body seriously instead of trying to placate or sedate it, is how much you discover about the levels of stress you operate under. Suddenly these levels become intolerable, which can mean you'll need to rest for longer or take breaks more frequently. This doesn't mean you become a good-for-nothing wimp, it means that you've stripped away a layer of numbness. Being fit will give you more energy, but if you're concerned with being fit and living well, you'll find it more difficult to tolerate circumstances that actually make you feel awful. What's surprising is how we do manage to numb ourselves into an impossible way of life that saps the body and drains the mind. In your present unhealthy condition you may want to argue that there is no other way for you personally to live. You're wrong. As you give yourself over to living well, you'll find imaginative and physical resources that allow you to dump the bullshit where it belongs. Where it doesn't belong is in your life. While you're having your early night and relaxing, think about things you'd like to do, trips you might make, people you want to get to know, anything in fact that frees your mind from its daily preoccupations. When you wake up the next morning, eat a fantastic breakfast, look in the mirror and decide that you're going to have a good day, whatever happens. Chances are, you will.

REASONS TO BE CHEERFUL ARE EIGHT

Just in case you're having a brief moment of panic and thinking that you can't change your life and even if you did what difference would it really make? I'm giving you a list of eight positive things that *will* happen if you decide you want to get fit and live well . . .

1 You will wake up in the morning to a body that's regenerated itself during the night. You won't wake up looking and feeling horrible.

2 Once you're awake, it won't take you half the morning to feel human because fitness means improved blood circulation. Your heart will be beating more strongly and distributing more oxygen to all parts of the body. That means vitality, you won't have to crank up the machine: you've got yourself a turbo.

3 You'll enjoy looking in the mirror. I always look in the mirror before I do anything else in the morning because it cheers me up. There you are, sleek and glossy, it's a confidence boost, especially if you reckon the day ahead might be difficult.

4 In or out of clothes, you look better. If you're not forced to be in the business of disguising your body you can wear almost anything you like, knowing that you won't be spreading out of the top or bulging out at the sides. Clothes become pleasure, not armour, and when you take them off in public or in private, you don't have to worry about what's underneath. Once and for all you'll end the tyranny of the wardrobe. Summer on the beach or by the pool is the ultimate ego trip.

5 People will admire your body and, interestingly, not in the sexist way that women are usually admired. A fine body is sexy, but it also commands respect. Respect and admiration can only do you good

6 Your sex life will improve beyond measure because you will become more desirable to yourself as well as to others. More secure and more energetic. When you feel more, you enjoy more, and when you're fit, you feel.

7   Mentally you'll be sharper and better able to cope with whatever comes your way. Everyone gets emotional and overwrought but you'll find valuable reserves of tact and strength that just aren't possible outside of a nourished, healthy body.

8   There's a certain extra power that comes with being healthy. An aura if you like that accompanies body confidence. It's a way of carrying yourself, a way of handling the world that's impossible to pin down and define, but it's noticeable and it works. Once you're in control of yourself, you start to control your circumstances.

So there we are. Isn't it time you took advantage of your own natural resources and made the most of yourself? If you've been reading this book so far with a certain amount of scepticism, I don't blame you. It's true that being fit and living well won't spirit away the mounds of washing up or the dirty cat litter, nor will tedium and boredom become automatically things of the past. Everywhere religion and quasi religion (under which heading I include the fitness package) are making claims on your soul and assuring you that all manner of things will be well, if only you believe. I'm not asking you to believe anything except that you are exceptional, and I'm not offering any solution you don't already possess. The energy and the determination are already there for the using. For a woman, physical confidence is in itself a change for the better. Behind every great man there's a tired woman and it's time we stopped making time for their greatness and made time for our own. I am convinced that living well in body and mind allows us to create for ourselves the kind of social and professional space we want. It's a mistake to think that driving ourselves into the ground is the only way forward. We have to work hard, and you'll have to work hard at getting fit and staying that way, but it's a different kind of endeavour to the soul-destroying grind a lot of us put up with in the name of personal progress. I am ambitious, but I know my ambition is better served by noticing every aspect of me and treating myself well. Your Grand Experiment will only take three months in the first instance, and if you don't think it's been worth it, then you stop. I don't think you will stop because the benefits long term and daily are too great, irresistible in fact. Being there is much more exciting than reading about being there, so why don't you find out for yourself?

CHAPTER 3

FUEL AND JUNK

If anything brought the twentieth century to its knees, it was instant coffee and an unnatural craving for sausages . . .

Food becomes us. Literally. Food converts into flesh and energy; into our substance and our output. If you don't eat well, don't expect to live well.

FATS AND FAT

Fats are a concentrated source of calories. You shouldn't allow your daily menu to contain more than 30 per cent fat. If you do, you're in trouble, not just because you'll add the pounds, but you run the risk of heart disease and skin problems. You should be especially careful with saturated fat which comes mostly from meat and animal products. It's not difficult to avoid fats once you get into the habit of recognizing where they lurk. Here's the danger list:

1 Red meat and mince in particular.
2 Rich cheeses like stilton, cheddar and boursin.
3 Creamy sauces.
4 Sweets, cakes, sausage rolls.
5 Butter and cream.
6 Fried foods of all kinds. Even the most innocent and fat-free food can be transformed into a fat-soaked mess. Anyone who fries spinach should be shot. Chips are not going to figure large in your life, and deep fried Camenbert should never get beyond a joke.

If you're eating out, approach the menu sensibly; go for a straightforward starter and follow it with a lean main course, like chicken or fish or something vegetarian. Have heaps of vegetables and salads and skip the pudding. At first you may find this hard, but after a few practice runs, you'll choose low-fat food automatically and enjoy it.

The annoying thing about fat is that whilst it comes into being through an excess of nutrients, it can't be changed back into those nutrients, meaning that your body still needs its daily supply of protein/minerals/carbohydrates etc. People talk about living off their fat, but this is a mistaken notion. The only real use for extra body fat is as fuel. So unless you're planning a long trip in a barren place there's no point carrying excess fat or eating excess fat in your diet. Western food is high on fat, but the daily dietary fat requirement for the average women is very small, and can be easily fulfilled without ever adding fatty foods to an otherwise balanced daily menu. Most foods contain some fat, even very lean meat; getting enough is the least of your worries. Fatty foods can't do anything for you except make you fat and generally out of condition. If you're storing fat, very likely it will be in the abdomen and thighs, so just remember that every time you go over what should be a modest fat consumption, you're sending the stuff right to where you least want it, and it's going to take a lot of hard work to get rid of it again. Every gram of protein that you eat contains four calories, every gram of fat that you eat contains nine calories, and bear in mind that whenever you eat a fat-soaked heavy meal and then go off to bed, your body can do nothing with that excess fat except store it. This is a pity, but it means that unless you're prepared to examine and alter the fat content of your diet, you'll have a hard time living well. A few intelligent changes, and you need never trip guiltily to the scales again.

THE TRUTH ABOUT SUGAR

Sugar is good for you in small quantities, and should only be taken pure and simple, in fruit or honey where the proportions are monitored by nature and the body can process it efficiently. The amount of sugar, and refined sugar at that, to be found in most pre-packaged sweet goods is too great for the body to use, and because it's refined, the body finds it more difficult to break down and redistribute. The fibre in fruit prevents the small amount of sugar present from entering the bloodstream all at once, but in packaged foods, there is no such barrier and so the body has to cope with an instant and usually overwhelming onslaught. This leads to the 'sugar rush', a brief surge of energy followed by a slump which means you feel tired and sometimes depressed. If you habitually pump excess sugar into your bloodstream, you will develop an abnormal craving for sweet things, one of the problems that binge-eaters experience. Like fats, sugars occur naturally in our foodstuffs, and unless you're planning to run a race or climb a high mountain in the cold, you don't need to be adding to the natural sources of energy. All you do when you take too much sugar is to throw your long suffering body mechanisms into a state of chaos which after a prolonged period can cause imbalances that are hard work to put right. It's not difficult to be on the side of your own body; all you need are a few facts and some determination not to give in to what the western world thinks of as convenient and pleasurable. If you have a sweet tooth, the best way to limit it is to go out of your way to eat sweet things that aren't artificial. Get involved in fruit. Exotic fruit so that you feel you're giving yourself a treat, and if you do buy chocolate, buy the most expensive kind. You'll be able to afford less of it and it will remind you of just how sickly those mass market yum yums really are. Taste is a matter of re-education, and if you give your body a chance it will start to tell you what you like and in what quantities. If cake is your Achilles heel, again buy the best, and try not to eat vast concoctions in restaurants. If you're at all dependant on any sugar product, you must try and alter that dependancy, because it means your body is out of true. I'm not implying that you can't eat cakes and biscuits and chocolate and ice cream and god knows what, only that these parts of your diet should be extras for occasions, not a daily deal. If you eat them on top of a normal diet, you're filling yourself with negative calories (calories you can't use) and forcing your body into a state of Red Alert as it desperately tries to accommodate sugar and fat it doesn't want.

HINTS

1 No sugar in tea and coffee. You'll get used to this quite fast and if you drink a lot of both, you can cut your sugar intake rapidly.

2 No point feeling self-righteous about the yoghurt if you buy sweetened fruit yogurt. Buy it plain and add your own fruit.

3 Watch out for sugar in tinned foods.

4 Go for mineral water rather than soft drinks. Your body likes pure water best of all, and it'll keep you well flushed out.

STARCH IS GOOD FOR YOU!

Starch is a complex carbohydrate i.e. an amalgam of simple sugars which break down steadily to provide your body with energy. If you eat enough starch, you won't have so much of a sugar craving, and you won't suffer the awful come-down that a sugar burn brings with it because carbohydrate actually releases a chemical in the brain called serotonin which makes you feel better. Clever! Getting and staying fat is not to do with starch, but to do with excess fatty and sugary foods. Starches are friends, so welcome them. You should eat starch food every day, wholemeal bread, cereals, potatoes, real pasta, pulses. Not only are these foods full of vitamins, they're also full of fibre and fibre is not present in many pre-packed convenience foods. You need fibre for your bowels and you should use it to keep your calories down, if you're an over-eater – fibre absorbs water and becomes bulky once inside you, so you don't feel you've got room for that cream bun. Fresh fruit and veg. are wonderful fibre sources and you'd do well to increase your intake of both and your intake of wholemeal bread. If you eat potatoes, which you should, get them in their jackets, the skin is packed with vitamin C as well as fibre. Try and eat rice and beans at least once a week. There's no point buying refined foods, especially when it comes to breakfast cereals, and then throwing your bran over the top. Buy muesli without added sugar, or construct your own cereal from rye flakes, oats, barley, plus fruit and wheatgerm. Wheatgerm is particularly good, and if you enjoy scrambled eggs, sprinkle some in just before they set.

POINTS ABOUT PROTEIN

Muscles, skin, hair, innards, bones etc. are made out of protein. We need protein to maintain this lot, but because the body is very efficient, we don't need much of it. Unfortunately our average diet is stuffed with it because it's particularly present in red meat and dairy produce, both of which tend to figure high in what people think is good for them. Better to get your protein (and you only need about 2 oz a day) from fish, white meat and vegetables. Red meats and dairy products both bring with them a large amount of fat.

VITAMINS ARE VITAL

VITAMIN A:
(Carotene)

This is toxic in excess because it's stored by the liver; however, it's unlikely that you're going to become so addicted to carrots and tomatoes that you'll poison yourself. This vitamin is best absorbed via red and yellow coloured veg., dairy produce and liver. You need it to maintain a glowing skin and good eyesight. So all those jokes about rabbits and carrots and sharp eyes had something at the bottom of them after all.

VITAMIN B
(complex)

Work together as a group, and one of their major functions is to keep the nervous system in good repair. If you live a stressful life you should consider your B intake as crucial because this complex can greatly reduce irritability, twitching, hysteria etc – an inadequate supply of B3 (Niacin) can cause mental disorder, and an inadequate supply of B6 (Pyrodoxine) will affect your dream life.

B1 (Thiamine), a nerve vitamin: this is lost from the body every time you pee and must be replaced daily.
B2 (Riboflavin): this helps you to resist infection and works with Vitamin A on skin health.
B3 (Niacin): a nerve vitamin and, again, related to skin health.
B5 (Pantothenic acid): a nerve vitamin. This one helps to produce the essential hormones that keep the balance between minerals and water in the tissues. Any kind of shock or emotional disturbance upsets these balances and leaves you feeling physically as well as mentally awful.
B6 (Pyridoxine): a nerve vitamin. Lack of this can cause irritability and stomach upset, and alcohol slows down its absorption. It's also known as the dream vitamin, and appears to play a major role in the chemical changes that accompany the dreaming state.
B12, a nerve vitamin: too little can cause anaemia.
Bc (Folic Acid): too little brings about disorder of the blood. It's sensitive to heat and is lost in cooking, so make sure you eat some leafy raw veg., (spinach salad is great) and treat yourself to oysters!

As you can see, the B complex is rather widespread in its effects,but fortunately it's easy to eat enough of it, if you think about your diet. Green veg., wholemeal bread, liver, eggs and grains will give you what you need, though if you're a heavy drinker, maintaining the B complex is one good reason to cut down. Probably you drink to combat stress but those stressful feelings are intensified by destroying the natural way of dealing with it. In effect you numb the nervous system because that temporarily makes you feel better, but what you're really doing is robbing your body of what it needs most when under stress. So go easy on the booze, and binge on green vegetables.

VITAMIN C

Easily lost in cooking, and certainly lost when you pee. Eat citrus fruit, at least one piece a day and if this makes you feel a prisoner, get a juice extractor and enjoy fresh orange juice for breakfast and mixed with champagne on long summer evenings (or even short winter ones).

VITAMIN D

The sunshine vitamin; which does not mean you will find it in cornflakes. This little number absorbs calcium which is the mineral vital to sound formation and reparation of the bones. You skin will obligingly soak it up from the sum, otherwise a couple of eggs a week is all you need.

VITAMIN E

Barbara Cartland's sex vitamin. Certainly it's connected with fertility and healthy blood cells, though whether it will turn you into a heroine of romance I don't know. It is astonishingly good for your skin, and I use it as a body lotion as well as eating foods that contain it. You'll find it in honey, wholegrains and wheatgerm and eggs, so those scrambled eggs with wheatgerm are going to set you up for a glowing weekend.

VITAMIN K

All we know about this is that it makes the blood clot and that we get it from leafy vegetables, so if you're eating properly you don't have anything to worry about.

Obviously this is the briefest trip around the vitamins and if you're interested you should read one of the books suggested at the end of this one. For women with particular deficiencies or illnesses, vitamins can make a vital difference and play a safer

role than drugs. If you do get overtired or myster-
iously depressed or find you suffer from nervous
rashes and headaches, it's worth going along to a
Nutritionist and having your diet properly checked.
Possibly all you are needing is a rebalance, which
means that drugs are unnecessary and that further
suffering is unnecessary too. What have you got to
lose but your pains?

**A WORD
ABOUT
CALCIUM**

Calcium deficiency is a serious nutritional problem
among women, and that's because women don't do
enough bone-stressing exercise and don't take care
of their calcium intake. You must get enough low fat
dairy produce and go for salmon which is full of
calcium and delightful to eat. Dark greens like kale
and broccoli are good too. If you don't get enough
calcium you're going to have a rotten (literally) time
when you get older, suffering from feeble bones,
bad teeth and hair loss. It's easy to make sure that
doesn't happen, but remember if you're already over
thirty-five you need to be especially watchful – your
body's at the stage where it needs more help.

THOSE PILLS

Only a variety of foods properly combined can give
you the full complement of vitamins and minerals
and too often vitamin pills are taken as a means of
avoiding dietary responsibility. It's part of the package
again – take this and all will be well. It won't. If you
eat badly you can pour pills down your throat till
nightfall and still look and feel like a slob. Forget
them and use your natural resources – good food
and common-sense.

**SHOCKING
SALT**

Most of us eat too much salt and this affects the
body's water balance. If there is a large amount of
salt knocking around in your system, your ever
faithful body will try and dilute it by retaining as
much water as possible. Result? Feeling bloated

which as you know is nasty and often depressing because it makes you think you're fatter. Here's what to do:

1 Use more herbs and spices and less salt in your cooking.
2 Remember that crisps and savoury snacks are full of salt.
3 Notice how much salt there is in packaged foods.

By now you will have realized that we add sugar, salt and fat to our diet quite unnecessarily, but as a matter of course. Understanding this will help you to stop doing it. For most of us the shortfall comes in the shape of fibre and essential starches. These are the things we need to concentrate on in order to live up to our bodies' potential. Of course the body is forgiving and it's clearly possible to go on functioning and eating thoughtlessly; we don't (not very often anyway) keel over in a heap, what we lose out on is *quality*. If we get used to under-living that condition will seem normal, and we will not link our aches and pains and depressions and niggly dissatisfactions with the way we are actually looking after ourselves.

THE DEMON DRINK

Don't worry, this won't turn into a lecture on temperance, and I'm applying the same principle to drink that I apply to everything else; buy the best you can afford. It's better for your body and your palate to enjoy one bottle of Chablis or Champagne than to consume a number of bottles of unlisted table wine. Similarly, if you like whisky, go for a single malt or a fine Bourbon. You may protest that you can't afford it, but probably you mean you can't afford to drink so much of it. Drink is best as a pleasure, not a prop. As we've already discussed, if you use it as an anaesthetic to combat stress, you're destroying some of the vitamins you need to counteract stress effectively. The other point is that alcohol enters the bloodstream quickly, rather in the way that sugar does, and so your body tries to use it as energy which, like too much sugar, it can't, especially as you're probably sitting down, or lying down, and are going to stay that way (sitting down uses a humble 1 calorie per minute). So what happens? You guessed it? – like excess sugar the body stores it in the fat cells. I could paint a horrible picture of a meal in a restaurant, and that meal is high on fat then you blow out on a huge dessert; meanwhile you slug away at the house wine then a few hours later you fall into bed with your fat cells bulging and your poor body desperately over-worked. Hangover? You should be dead.

THE NOT SO DEMON DRINK

Your body loves water; you're made up of at least 50 per cent water and you need to keep replacing it so that your tissues can bloom and your internal organs can be clean. If you don't drink enough water your body will hold onto what it's got with the desperation of a very large fish in a very small talk, which results in the condition known as water retention (often in the oddest of places). Getting your water via tea and coffee and soft drinks is not good enough; you need mineral water, at least a pint a day, taken straight and certainly first thing in the morning and last thing at night. For your body, which after all puts up with so much, this is such a pleasure, and it goes about its work rejoicing. If you've been drinking, you should try and consume the equivalent amount of water afterwards – otherwise you'll dry up, and feel lousy.

FAST FOOD FACTS

The best fast food you can eat is baked potatoes from those shops that offer them plain or with a variety of fillings. You get starch, fibre, vit. C, calcium if you choose cheese and B complex if you add salad, and you'd be pushed to go over 500 calories the lot. Burgers are popular, but the fibre content is low, mainly because they use such awful bread. Fat content is high and you could really overdose on sugar if you have one of the astonishing desserts burger joints tend to offer. Also, it's worth knowing that those skinny chips so loved by fast food joints everywhere have a higher fat content than thick 'chip shop chips' because you're getting a small amount of spud cooked in a large amount of fat. You could easily notch up almost 1000 calories with your burger/chips/dessert/drink, and if, as is often the case, you're eating your fast food late at night, where is all that fat going to go? Where is all that sugar going to go? Yes! straight into storage.

Fish and chips have been sneered at to some extent, and there is a tendancy to assume that they are more calorific and less nutritious than other fast food equivalents. This is not so. You end up with less overall calories than fried chicken and chips and less than a hearty burger meal. Certainly less than a doner kebab. Fish will provide calcium, peas will provide fibre, and the thicker chips, less fat and more starch. WARNING: don't cover the stuff with salt.

When it comes to sandwiches, you should choose wholemeal or pitta bread and low fat high energy fillings, especially if this is your lunch, because eating adequately will keep you away from the biscuit tin during the afternoon. Cottage cheese and pineapple, hard cheese and salad, tuna in brine and watercress, smoked salmon, plain chicken and tomato, plain egg and cress, will all give you a substantial meal, especially if you follow your sandwich with a piece of fruit, and drink water or fruit juice. Stay away from high fat fillings like salamis, corned beef, mayonnaise-mixed foods (tuna and egg) and watch against oily salad dressings. Increasingly popular and very good for you are wholefood takeaways like nut cutlets, aduki burgers, tofu burgers, nori rolls and bowls of mixed salad with such delicious things as alfalfa and bean sprouts. If you get hold of these things without too much effort, do so, not only because your body will love them, but because they allow your tastebuds to learn to do without sugar and salt signals.

THINGS YOU'D RATHER NOT KNOW ABOUT COFFEE

Caffeine has the same effect on your body as chocolate – both raise the blood sugar level very quickly, giving you the sensation of vitality that soon evaporates, leaving you tired, cranky, and wanting another cup. Chemically, it speeds up mineral loss, including that much needed calcium, and while it's doing that it produces acid in the stomach, which helps to make you feel tense and bad tempered. Pretty miserable eh? Then there's the problem of what accompanies those endless cups of coffee, cigarettes or biscuits, almost certainly something that makes your body feel like it's having a nightmare. If you like herb teas then you could drink those instead, or maybe substitute a couple of cups with mineral water or fruit juice, but it may be that the answer lies in the kind of coffee you drink. (I don't mean decaffeinated, that produces more acid in the stomach than ordinary stuff.) It seems to me that quality matters, food, drink, sex, clothes should all be a pleasure which is why I keep insisting that you buy less but buy better whenever you can. As far as coffee goes you can wean yourself off those mounting mugs of brown swill by determining that you will only drink freshly brewed Continental or Expresso – expresso strength in particular should cut down the need you have for caffeine because no one can physically drink that much of it, and it doesn't pretend to quench your thirst. It's thick and black and clearly there for another purpose. I never drink coffee when I'm thirsty but I do drink it when I want a shot of something potent. Your body can cope with and even benefit from most things in small doses and remember that expresso is very small, so a cup in the morning after your orange juice will set you up, and maybe another mid-afternoon or after your supper will give you the pleasant controlled high you want. That brown swill gives you nothing at all except undiscriminating taste-buds and an unhealthy desire for more of it. What's worse is that people usually think they've given their body the fluid intake it needs because coffee is largely water. Your body likes its water pure, it can use it better that way, and mineral water is much purer than anything you can hope for out of the tap. So drink plenty of spring water and enjoy your coffee as a stimulant, not a beverage. The Arabs wrote hymns in praise of coffee when they first discovered it; in my opinion it's a joy, especially because there are so many beautiful cups you can buy from which to drink it (small cups), and so many interesting gadgets to help you make it. It can be a hobby, though the worst insult is to percolate it or to accept it from one of those filter machines that allow it to stand and keep hot. Hot it might be, coffee it's not. Coffee should be fresh and pungent and full of the character of the moment. By the way, medically, it's classed as a poison.

WHAT ABOUT THE WEED?

You don't need me to tell you why smoking is bad for you: it causes cancer, bronchitis, emphysema, heart disease, bad breath, robs the body of vit. C and zinc, vital to skin repair (more wrinkles, faster) and leaves you vulnerable to illness and premature aging. It also makes exercise hard work and makes non-smokers suffer. If you want to live well, lay off.

DITCH THE DIET

This is a horror story. A true tale of terror for anyone who thinks that a diet is a good idea. If you go on a diet that doesn't give your body the nutrients it needs, it will look for those nutrients elsewhere, starting with stored glucose, but if it uses glucose to fuel its function then the water that always accompanies glucose has to go too – so it seems like you've lost weight, when all you've lost at first is water. When the stored glucose runs out, your body will start to manufacture it out of protein, which is hard work for your kidneys and liver and uses lots of water, which means that you'll have to drink more and then you'll start to feel bloated. As your diet continues the body will be unable to get on with its repair work and your muscles will start to shrink. You'll certainly lose weight, but too much of that weight will have been vital lean tissue that you've literally starved to death. That's why so many diets leave the unfortunate dieter with saggy skin and a strained gaunt look – without muscle there's nothing to hold you up! Your body hates the strain and will respond by creating more fat cells to store more glucose. Those fat cells are there to stay and that means you will put on weight quicker when you come off your diet. An all fruit diet will lose you lean tissue faster than anything except not eating at all, while all protein diets put too much strain on the internal organs. If you're overweight and do need to cut your food intake, you should seriously consider the content of what you eat before you start running for the cottage cheese and slimming biscuits. Probably you eat too much fat and too much sugar and that can be dealt with quite simply and efficiently as we've already discussed. Under no circumstances must you be seduced into a crash diet. If you're exercising, you need to fuel your body; the vital thing is to fuel it thoughtfully, so that you're helping the body build muscle and lose fat, not the other way round!

Our bodies are very sophisticated fat-storing machines because they're designed for survival and no one has yet found a way of helping them distinguish between a diet (less food because you want less fat) and a famine (less food therefore the body must hang onto its fat). Every time you diet your body gets worried and every time you stop your body resolves to make sure the crisis doesn't happen again and multiplies its fat cells and hangs onto whatever calories you give it because it thinks you're going to need them in the future. If you eat well and exercise frequently your body feels safe; it registers a regular input and output, gets on with its work and doesn't start altering its balance to cope with a chaotic world. Tiresome maybe, but that's the body you've got to live with. I haven't included a height/weight chart in this book because scales are inaccurate. Certainly they'll tell you how heavy you are, but they won't tell you the composition of that heaviness. They won't tell you what percentage of your body weight is water, what percentage is fat and what percentage is muscle. This is pretty useless as far as an accurate body assessment goes, and far too many of us get hooked onto the scales thing anyway. Two women of the same height and skeletal frame could stand side by side and one could weigh more than the other while still being a size smaller in clothes and looking a lot lighter – why? because muscle weighs heavier than fat, but muscle keeps the body in shape. You should be concerned with what your body's made of, not how heavy it is. Muscle tone makes a body look fantastic, and no diet can achieve it; diets in fact, as we've just seen, are likely to lose you more muscle than fat. Cutting your calorie intake by cutting out negative calories (excess fats and sugar) is not the same as dieting. I've heard women say they'd rather live on three Mars Bars than give them up in order to eat properly and lose weight. Madness, absolute madness; if we want to live well we have to work with our bodies instead of always expecting them to work for us and being surprised when they won't or can't.

BALANCED MEANS JUST THAT

A balanced diet is a diet that contains enough starch and protein and not too much fat and sugar. If you eat wholefoods and keep red meat for once a week, plenty of fruit and veg., and an eye on your dairy intake, there is no need to plan yourself a tortuous regime that adds to your guilt every time you fail to stick to it. Wash down your supplies with plenty of mineral water, be careful with coffee and alcohol and above all decide what foods you really enjoy (I'm hoping you won't say pastries, ice-cream, chocolate, sausages and very large helpings of steamed pudding) and eat them. You'll be surprised how many foods you like that are good for you. If your list does largely comprise fats and sugars, then you'll just have to retrain your palate, which is best done in sympathy with yourself, i.e. don't make huge mental and physical leaps from lots of sweet things to none at all, replace some of your sweet grabbing session with dried fruits or nuts and start to think carefully about what your body feels like before during and after your need for sweet things. If you tend towards cakes, switch to wholemeal scones that are packed with fruit, or eat fruitbread toast for breakfast and in the afternoon when you might be felled by a doughnut or waylaid by a rum truffle. It takes time to retrain your body if you've been stuffing junk down it for years but exercise will help to quell sugar cravings because it raises the blood sugar level and the body temperature (people want to eat less when they're hot). An extreme craving for sugars and/or fats may well mean you're badly lacking in starch and fibre and you should write down your average diet and analyse it in this light. If you don't see any imbalance, go to a Nutritionist and explain. It may well be, of course, that you're plain depressed, and the best thing you can do about that is to decide that you won't put up with it any longer.

As well as *what* you eat, balance is *when* you eat. Your body likes its food to come in regularly, it can process it better and it's less likely to have to store it in the fat cells. Small meals at regular intervals are preferable to two large meals, even though you might be consuming exactly the same amounts and the same sorts of food. Breakfast is vital. If you don't eat a proper breakfast, you'll be nibbling by mid-morning and your mental concentration will be less than its peak. You need energy when you start the day, so go for cereal and toast, or natural yogurt sweetened with fruit and honey, or baked beans or boiled eggs and as I already suggested, freshly squeezed orange juice and a cup of solid expresso. Oranges are not the only fruit, you could juicify almost anything that excites you. Fruit juice, though, does provide your body with vitamins and fructose (natural sugar) and obviously it's better for you if it's fresh rather than packaged. At weekends you could eat kippers and you could put champagne in your orange juice.

Lunch needs to be comprehensive; salad or veg., fish or white meat or one of my recommended sandwich combinations followed by fruit and washed down with mineral water. Drinking at lunch-time is not a good idea because it slows down the metabolism which means that you're less able in the afternoon, and it hinders your internal processing plant; your body, drowned in alcohol, can't deal with the food and deal with you, that's why you feel sluggish, the focus is on the inside, instead of what's going on at your desk. If you're on holiday, there's no reason at all why you shouldn't drink at lunch, but if there's work to do, it'll be harder, unless of course you've reached the stage where your body doesn't seem to function properly without booze . . .

Eating in the evening can be relaxed and generous, but it shouldn't be a heavy meal because usually you'll be going straight to bed afterwards and even the most energetic sex can't use up what you've just put in, so that leaves your body to go on working overtime, when what it would really like to do is have a rest. The later you eat, the more difficult it is for your body to process the food, because you have a body clock that expects a bit of peace now and again, and slows down accordingly. I never start eating after eight o'clock unless I'm doing something unusual that ensures I'll be able to cope with what I'm shovelling away. If it gets very late, like after 10pm and you haven't had your evening meal, it's actually better for your body to miss it altogether and wait for an enormous breakfast. If you're really ravenous then go for something light and easily digestible, like soup or a banana milkshake or a boiled egg. You aren't going to starve after all!

We all want to eat chocolate biscuits and cream cakes from time to time, and providing you usually eat exactly what you need and take care of your body, there's no reason not to. Similarly, too much booze now and again won't upset a healthy body. You're not about to live the life of a hermit; you're about to live better than ever before. Balance is not a once and for all condition, it's a continual readjustment to environment, personal needs and circumstances. Once you get used to listening to your body and understanding how best to nourish yourself and keep yourself in shape, you won't have any problem with indulgence, you'll indulge when you want to because wanting to won't be every day and it won't be in a way that's ultimately harmful. When you go on holiday, your diet will probably have to alter and you shouldn't care about that, if you're already healthy your body will adjust, though if you go to a place where the diet is particularly fatty and high in cholesterol, you should find out if there's anything else available. When in Rome etc., but when in America eat half of every plateful and refuse to have everything fried. Americans are excessively health obsessed, but they don't seem to be able to eat less food which is probably why they're so keen on stomach stapling. So pack your skipping rope and don't be afraid to say no. (According to Paul Ernsberger of Cornell: 'More Americans have died in the surgeon's war on fat than died in the Vietnam War.')

A WORD TO NIBBLERS

If you're a nibbler person, and you want to stay that way, take a long hard look at what your nibbles consist of. Crisps and peanuts will have to go. Chocolate bars too. You can eat fruit or wholefood snacks like Jordans bars, though you should remember that these do have a high calorie content, even though they'll keep you away from fat.

Nibblers have to make allowances for their nibbles. You can't eat a normal amount of food and have your snacks on top, not unless you're being very active. I suggest you try carrots. Carrots will do you good and after a time a combination of boredom and embarrassment will stop you nibbling altogether, which is much the best thing because the temptation to eat foods that are useless is at its most persuasive when it comes to nibbling. Obviously, if you're really hungry and it's not a meal-time and you can't get anything that looks remotely wholesome you're going to have to opt for peanuts. Make sure they're dry roast, and make sure you're not lying to yourself about that hunger pang. The trouble with nibbling is that it's often entirely unrelated to hunger. If you like to have a mid-morning or afternoon break, and you enjoy eating something with your cup of coffee, I realize that carrots are not the thing. Buy biscuits like Allisons or Brontë which at least use natural ingredients, and are higher in fibre and lower in sugars. The other trouble spot comes in the shape of nuts and crisps offered with pre-dinner drinks or at cocktail parties. Beware of Roka biscuits which are delicious but can leave you with a few extra pounds very quickly. If possible stick to olives, and if there aren't any olives refuse the rest. Nibbling is never very much at the time, but it adds up; if you don't believe me, make yourself a nibble list over a typical week and then work out both the calorie content and the fat/sugar ratio. You'll be surprised at least. Probably horrified.

BRAN?

Bran is not fairy dust. You can't sprinkle it over your food like a magic powder and hope it will at once regulate your bowels and give your body the fibre it needs. It's best to eat bran via foods that contain it, like wholemeal bread and cereal, otherwise there's a chance that it will actually prevent your body from absorbing certain minerals. The body likes synthesis and combination, it doesn't respond well to you stuffing things down *ad hoc* and hoping they'll all mix up on the inside and do you good. If you're constipated (which you shouldn't be on a healthy diet) then by all means ladle some over your breakfast, but don't be fooled into thinking that bran alone will solve your fibre and roughage problem. Too much of it will retain water and then you'll feel bloated. It's vital to understand that most of what we need, unless we have seriously depleted ourselves, is best found in our everyday food. Supplements are no substitute for a balanced diet, even organic ones like bran and wheatgerm. Use them sparingly.

TOOLS

You should buy a juice extractor and a blender so that you can make the most of fruit and skimmed milk drinks. If you buy new coffee making equipment, find the method you most enjoy and give yourself pleasure every time you grind the beans and prepare for a drink that in England revolutionized eighteenth-century intellectual life. When you appreciate your body, you'll want to fuel it with good things, and those good things can give your senses and your mind just as much nourishment as your body. Pans should be desirable as well as practical and if your crockery doesn't please you, throw it away and start again. Everytime you eat and drink you're celebrating as well as maintaining your life. Do it in style.

CHAPTER 4

GOOD AND BAD AT GAMES

Women have but one task, that of crowning the winner with garlands.

(Baron de Coubertin,
founder of the modern Olympic Games)

Women are more flexible than men.
Women are better balanced than men.
Women have more body fat than men.
Women adjust more quickly and more efficiently
to environmental change.
Women have greater long-term endurance powers
than do men.

Each of these statements is a positive statement, but did you wince when I mentioned the dreaded phrase 'body fat'? Probably you did, and that's because when women think about themselves in athletic terms they are usually thinking in male athletic terms. Women's advantages are different and separate and must be taken into account when considering the type of sport we might be better at or the type of sport we might most enjoy. Of course there are personal preferences, and women's individual bodies vary, but the basic points listed above are generally applicable.

FLEXIBILITY A woman's greater flexibility is largely due to a hormone called relaxin which operates most fully during pregnancy to widen the pelvic joints and the birth canal. It's also active during menstruation and present at a certain level every day which gives us an extraordinary degree of body mobility. Women then, should find it easier than men to stay supple or to regain suppleness even after periods of neglect. Relaxin also makes us better gymnasts, trampoliners, fencers, skiiers and martial arts experts – potentially, because of course all of those things need strength to match, but relative not absolute strength. Strength that is proportional to our bodies. Our flexibility gives us an advantage in those sports that demand style as well as strength, and where strength alone will not be the deciding factor in aptitude or victory. This is an exciting and understated attitude to sport. Too often women are not encouraged to consider their natural advantages and how to make the most of them, instead we're asked to focus on our disadvantages and how to overcome them.

BALANCE

Women have a lower centre of gravity than men much as do powerful motor bikes. This is mainly due to the female pelvis which is broader and shallower than that of the male. This makes us into balancers, we're harder to knock over, less likely to trip up and coupled with our flexibility keeps us the graceful stylish creatures we are – or should be. Interestingly, you may have noticed when you watch gymnastics that men don't do the Balance Beam at all. There are no competitions for them. Why not? Because they'd fall off! Men can't do it, but they don't like to tell us this. I always used to wonder why any coverage of the Balance Beam was always interrupted by the most macho of motor racing or wrestling, or boxing even more so than the normal gymnastic events which are still considered a bit effete unless the chaps can really ripple. Now I know. When women can't participate in a sport because of a physical consideration, that sport becomes particularly virile and worthy, like boxing. When men can't participate in a sport because their bodies aren't suitable, that sport is immediately marginalized. The same thing has happened with synchronized swimming. It's become a glamour sport for the girls, a sport that commentators can make sexist comments about and a sport that trivializes the very real *and female* skills in operation. Women are good at swimming because their extra pads of fat buoy them up and insulate them against temperature changes. Synchronized swimming demands the usual strength needed for swimming but it also demands flexibility and balance. It's an extremely arduous sport, men can't do it and they'd look ridiculous if they tried. Their bodies are wrong, but instead of admiring us women for succeeding at combining style and stamina they force it to the level of an aquatic Miss World and may the loveliest legs and the brightest smile win the day. It makes me want to kill.

I have a theory about limbo dancing. Who do you know that takes limbo dancing seriously? For most people it's a piece of tropical erotica certainly not worthy to be called a sport. But what's so different about leaping over a bar to inching under it? I'll tell you what. The high jump depends on explosive strength, which men are very good at because of their lower fat percentage, strong legs etc. Limbo depends on endurance (it takes longer) and balance and flexibility! What does this suggest to you? It suggests to me yet another instance where man can't bear not to be able to compete and, more importantly, win. I see no reason why limbo shouldn't be included as a legitimate Olympic sport providing we could persuade the commentators not to concentrate for too long on the shape of the competitors' breasts.

Women are good at moving beautifully and creating an aesthetic pleasure as well as displaying consummate skill in particular areas, but sport, because it is so much a male preserve, cannot bring itself to take aesthetics seriously, except in the non-macho sports like skating and gymnastics which none the less do their best to appear suitably manly (when men are performing) and suitably condescending when women take the floor. Consider the ridiculous frocks women wear on the ice rink as opposed to the men's matador style costumes which are sexy but virile. When it comes to the mat, men perform with steely eyed concentration and a powerful display of muscle while the women are required to cat walk about and curtsey and look as though they're playing at it. Which of course, as far as the men are concerned, they are. I think aesthetics in sport should be a major consideration, at least as important as the sweaty displays of strength that lie at the core of boxing, wrestling and weight lifting. If women are to experience equality as far as indoor sport is concerned, then the kind of things that we are good at, which aren't brute force activities, need to be given just as much coverage, prize money and status as the bullish games for boys. The same reasoning applies to snooker and darts, which women can be excellent at, and which at present, largely due to the nature of the competitors' stomachs and dress sense, is an extremely unaesthetic experience. It's taken women a long time to start to make any inroads at all into the preserves of the Working Men's Clubs – places where snooker and darts can be practised cheaply and with reasonable competition – but women are still excluded from major tournaments and the most likely spot to find a woman bending over a snooker table is still topless on the peanut cards behind the working men's bar. Reach isn't a problem, there are plenty of small fat men who play snooker and still manage to squash themselves over the table; balance and flexibility certainly aren't at issue, and it doesn't take an inordinate amount of strength to hold a cue or a dart. The issue is the usual one: sexism. Women can't because women can't. So if you feel you want to play snooker then gather some women friends about you and brave the inevitable insults and bum pinching that will follow. It won't keep you fit as such, but the anger you'll experience will burn off a few calories and you're saying that women can, can do it well and can do it with style.

BODY FAT

Don't skip this section, it's interesting. Women have a considerably greater percentage of body fat than do men, an average percentage for a woman in her twenties would be 23–30 per cent, below 20 per cent periods would probably stop and she would feel the cold acutely. For a man of the same age, even 23 per cent fat would be a bit on the flabby side, and 12 per cent would not be an unusually low level. At a similar level a woman would be heading for big trouble. We need our extra fat which is why aiming for a body that looks like a man's is not only stupid but dangerous. What matters is to keep our fat level at a fit level. Without a computer it's difficult to determine how much of a person's body is fat, so if you have a gym that will do a computer reading, go along and find out what you are. On the other hand it's easy to tell whether or not you're actually carrying around too much fat – mainly because you pop out of clothes and because it gets in your way.

Body fat looks different on men and women because it's stored in different places; men carry it largely over their abdomen, which is why they get pot bellies while keeping relatively slim hips. Women store it around the thighs, hips, bust and behind the arms (the place where our triceps are supposed to be) but not especially on the stomach. The reason many women have rounded stomachs is because the stomach muscles aren't tight, not because women are necessarily overweight. This extra body fat is obviously a disadvantage in sports that require the body to propel its mass, which is why men tend to excel at jumping and running, though trained women are catching up. What bothers me is that women's bodies might become like men's bodies if we're required to participate and perform in the same way that they do. This remark lays me open to obvious criticism because it's precisely the argument that men have always used, except that they've used it to argue their own superiority, i.e. that a certain shape (the male shape) is the ideal shape for athletics and that women will have to become quasi-men and find themselves unable to compete against men – and win. My argument is that athletics has been designed around the male shape and designed to suit male skills and, as I suggested earlier, the only sensible approach is to stop the hierarchical grading of sport so that only 'manly' sports receive proper attention and rewards. We have already noted that women are better than men at endurance activities, because they have less explosive (instant) strength than men, but more stamina, and this stamina is because they have more body fat which can be broken down slowly into fuel at the same time as protecting the body from upsetting changes in temperature. What does it matter if women don't beat men over short distances when they are adept at marathons and proving that their fastest time will soon be faster than the men's? In swimming body fat is an advantage because it buoys up and insulates. Women hold most of the long distance swimming records including the single and double channel swim. Women's bodies are different but they are not second rate. They excel at different things and those things need proper recognition. Women also need the confidence to develop their bodies along their own lines, not on some spurious male model. Unless you want to attack your body fat in a way that will make you ill or at least affect your female functioning rather dramatically, you would be better to rejoice in your positive advantage of more fat and have a look at some of the exciting endurance activities that, coupled with your greater balance and flexibility, put you ahead of the boys straight away. We don't have to do it their way, it's just another aspect of their paranoia that when they discover they can no longer ignore us (because we demand the right to sport) they set about trying to absorb us, and that often means coaching us into bodies we can't use to the best of our natural advantages. I'm not suggesting you shouldn't run and jump and power lift and whatever you want, only that you shouldn't judge yourself on explosive strength, or indeed absolute strength at all; you need relative strength, the strength that suits and powers your own body. Do they get upset because they can't do the balance beam? or the limbo pole? or synchronized swimming, or long distance swimming? No. For the boys, macho is still mucho, but for my money, balance, flexibility and endurance skills have just as much to offer.

WOMEN AND CHANGE

Women adjust to changing environmental conditions more quickly than men, which may not sound like a very useful skill outside of a crash in the desert, but is in fact extremely useful if you want to try running at altitude, trekking through foreign parts, or even buying a mountain bike and scudding round the mountains. And of course, there's adventure sailing which women have always been involved in, though usually minimized by the press as cleaners or tea makers or any of the other adjunct things that men need when they go on a trip. Women are at an advantage over men in humid conditions because we lose heat via radiation rather than via sweat (one reason why women go red in the face). This keeps us cooler and it means we conserve vital amounts of water. Our bodies are altogether less badly affected by increases or decreases in temperature, not just because we have more of that fat but because of our periods. Yes, they have another use besides babies – our menstrual cycle in fact accustoms our bodies to temperature change every month, so really it's no big deal when the environment does it as well – so if the boys say you can't get in your Landrover and see the world, tell them to get stuffed – if anyone's going to faint and complain, it'll be them. What with our balance and our endurance and our acclimatization we should be mountain climbing and pioneering, not sitting in the jeep doing map references.

**ENDURING
WOMEN**

Women endure. You knew that anyway. We are much better at enduring than we are at sprinting or using our explosive strength and again this is because of the way we're made. Men's blood contains more haemoglobin – an oxygen carrying chemical, which allows more oxygen to be made available more quickly when the muscles need it – this gives them a greater aerobic capacity (this and their larger heart and lungs) – so men are better at getting the power going fast and using it efficiently. For women, the process is slower and steadier and this, coupled with the fact that women convert their fat into fuel once the glycogen in the muscles has been used up, contributes to their slower sprinting and short distance times and their greater relative and soon to be absolute ability on long distance track times. Already, their swimming endurance is superior. You may not know that women prove extremely reliable and usually unbeatable when it comes to flying records. Women appear to be able to stay awake longer, to manage on interrupted sleep (probably because of babies again) and to concentrate more totally than do men. However, women's flying records are always minimized and usually only mentioned during the rapturous applause that follows every time the boys win one back. Women have been continually dismissed as rally drivers on the grounds that they're too feeble to deal with the hardship, whereas our bodies deal with that kind of hardship far more efficiently than do men's.

**MORE BODY
FACTS**

Luther noticed that women have broader hips than men and concluded, in the way that only men can, that this meant we should sit on them and push children out of them; obviously he didn't know how useful it is to have a lower centre of gravity, but then he'd never ridden a powerful motor bike. When it comes to shoulders, men definitely show a muscle advantage and build strength quite quickly over the back and chest without really trying. For women, building muscle here will take time. Our muscle power is similar in strength to men's, but men have more of it. The extra upper body power of males plus their longer and differently shaped arms gives them a distinct advantage when it comes to throwing and racket games. A man's arm, held straight out makes a clear line, whereas a woman's shows a definite angle at the elbow joint. there's no question that these differences affect game aptitude. Shape and strength explain why, for instance, so many men could beat Martina at tennis. They are capable of a much more ferocious serve and of returning the ball at speeds which women simply can't match because our arms are shorter, differently shaped and can't be propelled by the same amount of chest, back and shoulder power. Women used to play tennis their own way, and the kinds of games offered by male and female players were quite stimulatingly different. I don't think the streamlining of the game makes it more interesting, and it certainly doesn't make it a fairer contest. Streamlining nearly always means doing it the male way, and as we're finding out, women aren't designed to do it the male way. Pointing out that we're built on other lines isn't asking for a soft option; it's expecting to be treated as equals but treated as women instead of becoming some kind of androgny at best, male clone at worst in the world of mixed sport. Again this is open to misinterpretation; women have had to fight against male ideas of what we can and can't do, and certainly women's body training schemes often teeter between the coy and the condescending as the male instructors try to decide what to do with what they see as a rather inferior specimen. I believe that women should involve themselves in very vigorous weight, aerobic and endurance activities and that we should choose to explore any sport we like, but I also am convinced that we need more intelligent challenging of the whole sports ethos which seems to me to be primarily male – there are only three women for instance and eighty men on the Olympics committee. We may have forced men to include us, but we're still letting them make too many decisions for us, and muscle power and how to channel it is still the focus of most sporting activity because that suits men's bodies best. Women have periods – men don't – therefore periods are seen as a sporting disadvantage rather than as part of a sporting cycle that allows the body to function in other than in purely mechanical ways. Gloria Steinham has written a wonderful piece in her book *Outrageous Acts and Everyday Rebellions*, called 'If men could menstruate' and she says wittily and rightly, that if men could they'd make it into a status symbol and incorporate it into their virile mythology (which would inevitably mean incorporating it into sport) it would be a rite of passage into adulthood, they'd boast about how long and in what volumes (I'm a three pad a day man) and they'd probably all hope and pray they timed it right for the day of the big race. Whatever they did with it, they wouldn't call it a handicap, because men don't have handicaps (despite the fact that they fall off the balance beam) they have advantages and bigger advantages. Women's bodies are not 'unreliable' they are subject to change in a way in which men's are not, and in a way that, as we have seen, gives them positive plus points when it comes to acclimatizing and conserving fluid (vital for any distance exercise). If men could menstruate they would accuse women of having static bodies – bodies that lacked internal co-ordination and bodies that were unable to cope with change. Because they can't they call their own bodies reliable – ours wayward, theirs, the model. We don't have to accept this. They fashion their lives around their salient points – why shouldn't we expect to do the same? Might is not right, it's just noisier.

WALKING AWAY

In the comments that follow on various kinds of sporting activity for fitness, pleasure and competition, I'll be focusing on our advantages and how to get the best out of ourselves. If we're going to live well, we're going to have to make the most of everything we've got. You may not think that walking sounds very dynamic, after all you do it each day. But it's a mistake to confuse the familiar with the dull. Walking, like most usual things, is as exciting as you want to make it. We're responsible for our own enjoyment, so we might as well start by enhancing the basics. An efficient walking technique will help to keep you fit and could become your major out of gym activity. Brisk walking raises the pulse, so it's aerobic and it greatly strengthens the muscles in the legs, buttocks and lower back. Women are naturally fine walkers, because of our lower centre of gravity, our better balance and our naturally strong legs – just as men have the advantage in the upper body, women have the advantage down below. Men have absolutely longer legs, but women usually have longer legs relative to their body proportions. Our power lies here, so let's use it. Walking isn't a pounding action in the way that running is; it's gentle, rhythmic and controlled. It places a very healthy stress on the bones, and that's a stress we need along with a sufficient calcium intake, to maintain our skeleton in peak condition. It is the lack of bone stressing exercise that causes osteporosis in women (brittle and easily broken bones in later life). Walking uses more of the muscles more of the time than almost any other sustained activity and it's hard on the fat – walk briskly for around two hours and you've lost over 500 calories, walk uphill and you'll lose even more. In the States more and more people are walking to work, claiming it makes them feel alert and relaxed before they have to deal with the pressures of the day. Certainly, if you've decided that the only real space you can find for yourself is early in the morning then the best fitness and overall well-being training plan you could perform would be to get up, wander about and drink your orange juice, do your stretch exercises, eat breakfast then walk to work, or a distance towards work that is comfortable and fits in with your daily schedule. If you did this, and managed a couple of workouts a week at the gym – preferably not first thing – you would soon experience great changes in your mental and physical states. For anyone who has decided to go all out on the gym business, walking is still a wonderful supplement and one that you can only benefit from. All you need to do, is put your head up, feel your spine straight and use the whole power of the foot as you walk, heel to toe in a controlled rolling motion. Breathe deeply and fully and let your arms swing back and forth. You should be walking from the hips, not from the thighs or knees and you should use your whole body. Using your whole body is very sexy anyway, and will improve your life in other areas.

Footwear is obviously very important, especially since a lot of women have caused themselves an abnormal shortening of the calf by wearing high heels. If you really have been a high heel freak for years, then flat shoes are going to feel very uncomfortable at first, but they're going to have to become a feature of your new fit self, whatever you decide to take up, so walking might be a good initial way of breaking you in. I know that Jack Lemmon and Tony Curtis did wonders in heels when they starred with Monroe in 'Some Like it Hot', but if you can manage to avoid chasing through hotel lobbies in your pinkies or even walking any distance at all in shoes that are actually designed for something that isn't in fact the female leg but the fetish leg, you'll be doing yourself a favour. No need to abandon heels, just wear them with care. Walking shoes should allow plenty of room for the toes, should never pinch at the sides or rub at the heel. Go to a good sports shop or specialist running shop and tell them your intentions and be prepared to pay for what you want: £25 is average. Don't forget you'll be wearing socks, so you might need a bigger size than you think. It's best to take a pair with you. If walking carries you away, you'll need to invest in a couple of pairs, so that you're not always treading in the old sweat before it's had time to evaporate. Women are used to walking; it's a feature of our lives – taking kids to school, shopping, all the fetching and carrying that still comes with being female. If we do it, we might as well make sure we're doing it to serve ourselves as well as other people. For women who don't have to walk much – it's time to start again. Leg muscles are woman muscles and you'll be pleased to know that the extra fat we carry on our hips is again an advantage when it comes to race-walking which is different to ordinary walking in that the hips must rotate fully at every stride. Rotating is easier for us than lifting our body mass off the ground, which is what happens when we run. In addition, race-walking is an endurance activity and like all endurance activities burns off the calories. So it's up to you, you can walk briskly for general health and enjoyment, or you can use your natural advantages even more fully and get involved in race-walking. I have included a list of contacts at the end of this book.

THE HARE AND THE TORTOISE

Running is not just moving at a different pace to walking, it's a whole different activity because it's really a series of leaps where the body leaves the ground. Walking involves a rolling motion not a leaping motion. The first thing to think about when you're wondering whether or not to run are your feet. Women don't have the same shape feet as men, so don't be beguiled into buying any of the (cheaper) unisex shoes still on the market. A woman's foot has a narrower heel and instep than a man's so while you may find that a multi-purpose model fits you, you will also find, surprise surprise, that it has been designed for him not her and won't give you the support you need around the ankle. Running shoes need to be just that – shoes for running, don't use them for anything else, and don't try and get away with wearing your all-purpose training shoes. You only get one pair of feet, so you must look after them. Another important point, if you're not used to choosing track shoes, is that they don't become more flexible with time, only more worn. So remember that they have to feel comfortable when you first wear them in the shop, and you can't extend their life. They'll wear out according to how much you use them and that's that. If you have breasts that need support, don't start running without investing in a non-chafe sports bra with cotton sides, otherwise you may find that sweating leads to soreness and even the dreaded jogger's nipple. If your sports shop doesn't stock sports bras, complain (and then go to Marks & Spencer, who do). When you decide to run, remember your advantages as a woman – that you are going to build your endurance levels, that you are especially competent at long distances and that your body is tolerant of temperature change, which makes you a good candidate for hill and dale running in all weathers. Don't worry about speed to start with, enjoy the movement of your body and take yourself as far as you can without real pain:

1 Warm up before you run, a few stretch exercises for ten minutes will do.

2 Wear the right shoes and light loose clothing that will absorb sweat.

3 Pick a route you enjoy, and change it when you don't.

4 Take account of your times and improve your distance/time ratio slowly.

5 Measure your pace, you should be able to hold a conversation and run.

6 Land heel first and push off with the ball of your foot.

7 Concentrate on running upright and keeping your legs straight.

8 As you end your run, slow down to a walking pace, regain normal breath and do some more stretch exercises before you decide the effort's over.

If you're overweight, smoke a lot, have a heart condition or are over thirty-five and not used to exercise at all, don't start vigorous running without having a check-up . . . it's not worth the risk. If you find you enjoy running, and a lot of women do because it's a flexible sport that allows independence and builds body confidence, then you'd do well to meet up with other women and involve yourself in group or club activities. Running with a friend is stimulating and you can spur each other on when it rains or one of you wants to watch 'Chariots of Fire' instead. Company staves off despair, and certainly there'll be some days when you'll wish you'd never started. If you like it, you'd do well to enter fun runs and marathons as soon as possible. It doesn't matter if you don't finish, it's an important feeling of team togetherness that men get a lot of and women miss out on. Check the contacts at the end of the chapter and good luck!

WATER ON THE BRAIN

Women and water is a powerful combination. If you swim a couple of times a week for as little as half an hour your body will improve. That is, you will become stronger, sleeker and probably want more exercise. Your pads of extra fat will support you, and although swimming is largely reliant on the upper body to power you along, because your mass is supported by the water, it's less of a burden on those underused muscles and a speedy way of strengthening your back and shoulders. Women tend to be timid in the water at first. Consider any pool and its occupants – the men beat along, usually using crawl or backstroke or some other stroke that splashes all over the place, while the women, heads out of the water, do a neat little breast stroke. Why women have become breast stroke addicts, I don't know, at least not the nice breast stroke. If you're going to do it at all, your head should be under the water for half of the stroke, and your shoulders raised right out for the other half, that way, you use the muscles involved to their full capacity, as well as forcing the heart and lungs to work strenuously and rhythmically. If you're a poor or timid swimmer, you should take lessons, bearing in mind that you have natural advantages that you can capitalize on. Women can build ability in the water as soon as they clear their heads of preconceptions about being fragile or weak. A woman who knows how to use herself in the water is about as weak as a double decker bus, and that applies to all women, especially overweight ones who will find that being supported by the water is an absolute boon, allowing them an exercise freedom they couldn't hope to achieve on dry land. The way to get the most out of swimming is to vary your strokes, so that most of the body gets used during your session. A combination of forceful breast stroke, energetic crawl, powerful backstroke and possibly some butterfly when your shoulders improve, will not only put you in peak condition, it will also clear you a lane in the pool.

Swimming is one of the best natural relaxers available, better than booze or pill and on a par with good sex. What's more it relieves back ache because our bodies get fed up with standing up and if you're already feeling the pinch, lying down won't help but a swim will. Moving your body without the weight of gravity gives it a chance to stretch, freeing trapped muscles and revitalizing tired joints. It's a tonic as well as a workout.

If you hate chlorine, all I can suggest is that you wear goggles to protect your eyes and swim very vigorously for not too long. Regular pool swimming demands conditioner for your hair, and thorough showering followed by a penetrating body lotion to prevent skin and hair from drying out and flaking. If you live near an outdoor pool or can get to the sea (in season) this is obviously much better for you; fresh and salt waters are beneficial on the skin and will give you a glow that a pool cannot.

If you decide to take swimming lessons, why not learn to dive at the same time? Diving is an interesting mental discipline because you must picture your body at a certain angle and project that picture of yourself into the water. Done well, diving is aesthetic and exhilarating – done badly, you look like an off balance frog. But women again have an advantage – our lower centre of gravity which allows us to project cleanly and gracefully into the water, once we understand the basic technique. When it comes to somersaulting and flipping through the air we have all the bonus points; our extra mass is in the air, so we don't have to lift it; we're flexible, balanced, and the only strength we need is strength that is proportional to our bodies. The only barrier is in our heads – it's a sport that suits us because we're women, not a sport we have to teach our bodies to adapt to outside of their natural skills.

PEDAL POWER

Cycling will pump up your heart and lungs and burn around 300 calories an hour. It firms your legs, tummy, shoulders, arms and back and it doesn't put any strain on the joints. It doesn't matter how out of condition you are, you can cycle at your own pace, stop if you want to, and experiment with little bursts of speed during an otherwise leisurely run. Even if you do lots of other exercise, cycling to work can only improve matters and if you live in a city, the bike will probably get you there faster. Needless to say, the type of bike you ride is of the utmost importance. Old gearless bikes are best kept in the shed. You need a bike that is sturdy, lightweight, the right size, properly geared and properly balanced if you're going to carry loads as well as yourself. A three speed straight handle bar job will enable you to cruise around quite happily, but it won't really allow you to work on your performance. If you want to strengthen and empower your body, you need a machine to work with you, not to make the whole thing more of an effort. It's a mistake to think that because a bike's harder to pedal, it's doing you more good. If that were the case, athletes would all ride around on bone shakers. Racing bikes are geared to help you make the most of the terrain and your legs and to regularize your aerobic capacity. The faster the wheels go round, the more you are exercising your muscles; a bike isn't a piece of weight training equipment to strain against, the important thing is to keep the wheel turning – 75 revolutions per minute is a steady speed, going up to 100 as you feel fitter and more confident. Straining in too high a gear or on a grotty bike tires you out, gets you nowhere and because we're women, can strain our knee joints. Racing bikes are the most sensible and versatile things you can buy, whether you choose a cross bar or one of the excellent women's frames around makes no real difference. Drop handlebars allow you speed and control, make your body more streamlined and take the weight off the bum. They also allow you to shift position, which on a long run is very necessary. Remember that you can have two sets of brakes fitted onto the handlebars so that you can ride in the upright position if you choose. If you do buy a crossbar bike, make sure the saddle suits you. Boys are again built differently around the crotch, as you've probably noticed, and what feels comfortable for them might not feel so good for you. When you go for your test ride, make sure you can live with the saddle and if not get the shop to change it for you. I'm a believer in toeclips – they're safer – your foot can't slip off the pedal but you can free yourself very easily if you want to, and they allow you to make the most of the pedalling movement. A lot of women claim they feel unsafe using them, but it just takes a little time and a few practice runs. If you're cycling to work you need a bike that can cope with traffic, which racing models can, and as far as I'm concerned, uprights can't. They don't have the versatility to cope with the usually awful conditions experienced around car drivers. Women on bikes is another healthy combination, because our leg muscles give us immediate power while cycling itself builds the weaker area in the upper body and abdomen. It's also the sort of activity you can do when you feel like it, and the sort of activity that you can use for your own purposes, without feeling embarrassed at being less good than someone else. When bicycles were invented they allowed women a previously unknown freedom and we designed the bloomer to cope with it. Nowadays the bloomers have gone, but the freedom is still there – freedom to go when and where you want and know that it's keeping you in good shape at the same time. Like running and walking, cycling can be an individual or a communal activity, depending on what you enjoy. Why not go away with a friend for the weekend, take the train and hire a bike to take with you. That way you'll have an adventure, and adventures are good for us, and you *can* decide whether or not cycling suits you.

MAKING A RACKET

If you enjoy competition, rather than group or individual activity, then racket games are a good idea, allowing you to improve and be encouraged by playing people who are better than you are. Tennis and badminton use between eight to twelve calories a minute, depending on how hard you play, and can be played by anyone with some enthusiasm, even those who are not especially fit. Like other sports you should warm up before you hit the courts. If, however, you're looking for a game that keeps you in peak condition at the same time as developing your powers of concentration and drawing out your innately savage qualities (which may help women to be more assertive in other areas) you should try squash.

Squash isn't a game to get fit on, it's too arduous, using a wide range of muscles to their full capacity and burning up to twenty calories a minute. A thirty-minute game will give you a total aerobic and stamina building workout, though it should be remembered that if you can run comfortably for thirty minutes off the squash court, you're not really up to playing for thirty minutes on it. Not many women play squash, perhaps because of the physical demands, perhaps because it can be expensive (court and club fees tend to be higher than for other sports), but most clearly, I think, because it's been appropriated as a male preserve. Women who do play and want to play well complain of sexism and violence when they join a league or a club. Men don't take them seriously and if a woman shows particular prowess, she's often offered a much more violent game than is necessary. We're back to the physical thing again in that men have longer arms, stronger bodies and so play a different game to that of the women. Typically they are unable to adjust to a woman's game and demand that she adjust to theirs, which can be very uncomfortable, not to say dangerous. Women who start to play should do their best to find a woman coach and, if possible, other women of varying standards to play with. Sometimes the best thing you can do is to advertise if no one you know is available. Anything's preferable to playing against men in the early stages of your development. If it's any consolation, experts agree that women play a more interesting game, because we have to rely on tactics and skill, whereas men tend to rely on muscle power, whopping the ball all over the place and not concentrating on the zen of placement. Obviously men who are good play well, but women have to depend on playing well from the start because they don't have that power to help them out. Men just hit their way out of trouble, women have to be clever. When you become an exceptional squash player you might have a lot of fun playing men, but until then, you're more likely to find it boring and dispiriting – they won't accommodate you, you'll have to return ferocious balls that belie the skill of the game, and you won't get much chance to improve. Leave them to it, and persuade a friend or friends to share your enthusiasm. Women I have spoken to who play squash regularly tell me it sharpens their overall concentration and decision making abilities, and it does seem to be a way of focusing mental and physical skills into a desirable whole that has benefits outside of the game. Women find it difficult to express their anger, especially when dealing with stubborn and/or stupid male colleagues, so it may well be that the nature of the game allows more rage to be comfortably released at the end of the day than is otherwise possible, at the same time as reasserting a woman's prowess and various abilities. Squash involves thinking very rapidly and staying one move ahead, skills which women need to succeed and which can be developed on court. It may well be that men have noticed the kind of edge, mental and physical, that squash allows, and that women are better tactically even though they can't compete with men physically. In a society that's rapidly ruling out brute force as the deciding factor in technological and professional success, men have every reason to worry that women's skills are going to be more appropriate. Not surprising, then, that wherever they can, they reinforce strength as the issue, even in a game like squash where there's no absolute sense behind it at all, only a relative whim, because as long as the game's about strength, they can win. For you as a woman the game is about skill. Learn it on court and use it wherever you need it.

FIGHTING FIT   The martial arts are non aggressive but they are assertive which is what makes them so suitable for women. Women can use their natural abilities to the full; their sense of balance and timing, their flexibility, even their extra fat which acts as a comfortable cushion to break the inevitable falls. Most important, women who learn the martial arts learn that instant and greater muscle power isn't the key to winning. A trained women can defend herself successfully against an untrained man, and against a trained man will still find herself on a level of realistic competition. Her lower centre of gravity will ensure that she has a better chance of staying on her feet, too! Unlike most western sports, the martial arts are concerned with the harmony of body and mind, the utilizing of all the resources towards a single end. This means time and practice and perhaps because women are encouraged to be patient they make more disciplined pupils than do men. As far as fitness goes, you'll enjoy the martial arts to a greater degree if you already have some effort behind you. They're strenuous, placing a lot of emphasis on the legs and back and using anything up to 400 calories an hour, so if you're hoping to use them to actually get fit, you've a lot of pain ahead and you'd be wiser to undergo a training programme for a couple of months first.

Judo meaning 'the gentle way' is the most popular of the martial arts. It's due to be featured for women as well as men in the 1988 Olympic games which should be a very interesting insight into male/female techniques of a non-combative sport. Judo depends on using the attacker's own force to disarm her or him by a series of overbalancing wrestling grips.
Aikido, 'the way of all harmony', depends on holds, locks and throws rather than on wrestling grips and because the joints are the main targets here, expect soreness and stiffness for a while, though women will loosen up more quickly than men because of their levels of relaxin (see p. 69). Essentially aikido is an aesthetic art, the object being almost to dance with your partner as you seek to overcome them.
Tai Chi, Great Ultimate Fist is probably the most suitable of the martial arts for women who are older or who have any joint disability like rheumatism. Its slow undemanding pace, makes a good toner and strengthener whatever your stage of fitness, while the slow repetitions induce a sense of peaceful relaxation at the same time as increasing balance and improving breathing. You might even find yourself in touch with the energy of the universe that the Taoists believe can be tapped via Tai Chi.

Women who get involved in the martial arts tend to stay keen and progress quickly and our numbers are growing, so you won't have any trouble finding a club with a good proportion of women members and the kind of tuition that helps women specifically. It's not a sexist sport either, probably because the emphasis can't be placed on biological body strength. Men and women can compete together in a way that proves satisfactory to both parties and the audiences at formal competitions seem to be genuinely mixed. For women the martial arts are a non-threatening high reward activity that isn't very expensive and does provide a great deal of personal confidence within a team environment.

SNOW ON YOUR BOOTS

Skiing is exhilarating, terrifying, tremendous fun and a first rate aphrodisiac. It's also a marvellous all over body toner and you as a woman with strength in your legs and a good sense of balance should be good at it. The thing is, though, you can't be unfit and hope to ski, so why not decide right now, that after your initial three months get fit trial, you'll give yourself a skiing holiday, providing of course you maintain your new purposeful self until the time it's best for you to go. Fitness opens a whole heap of new things to do and you do everything so much better, but skiing for me is one of the real pleasures that can only be fully appreciated through a healthy body.

There are two types of skiing, downhill and cross country. Downhill will call on your strength, co-ordination and general flexibility, though not much on your heart and lungs, while cross country is just about the most demanding thing you can take up. You can't rely on the slope to get your speed going, you have to propel yourself using almost every muscle you possess and a dose of will power besides. As a consolation you will burn up 800 calories an hour if you put your back into it. If you fancy cross country, then make sure that your training programme includes weights, you can be as supple as you like but if you haven't got enough power in your shoulders, you won't get very far – obviously men have an advantage on cross country because they've already got the muscle by design, but don't worry, they also have denser bodies that need more muscle to move them about. If you're strong in proportion to your frame, you won't have any problems whisking yourself along. If you've never skiied before, you might like to get used to the feeling by learning down hill, where you won't need so much body power up top. Not only will you return looking better and glowing all over whether you choose cross country or downhill, you'll be convinced that all your fitness efforts weren't in vain and go back to your workouts with new enthusiasm.

BOUNCING HEALTH

For women who are large or unfit or feeling that their bodies are ungainly, trampolining can be the perfect way to find the impetus you need to train and enjoy your body. Size and previous experience don't matter at all on a trampoline and if you're used to feeling that your body's too heavy, imagine the triumph and pleasure you will experience as you fly through the air. Trampolining courses are readily available in most towns at the local sports centre or YMCA and enthusiasts are growing in numbers, particularly women. It's a very good natured sport where everyone makes a fool of themselves for a while without a sense of incompetence. You're learning to control your body in a completely different environment – the air – and that demands a fresh approach, the kind of approach that many women have, perhaps because they don't have the same amount of inbuilt ideas about sport as men do. If you haven't used your body fully for a long time, trampolining will give you an all over sense of yourself, because you can't throw one bit in the air without throwing all of you along with it. You will develop co-ordination, grace, and an understanding of how your body is actually weighted when gravity isn't intervening. Male and female bodies are obviously weighted differently and so the balancing process on the trampoline is not the same. You'll get a fascinating sense of how you work and how they work, just by watching men and women use the trampoline in a way which suits them. As your confidence grows you'll find yourself moving differently off the trampoline as well as on it because you'll have an interior mirror picture of how your body holds and directs itself. Any activity that makes you feel good about your body will promote weight loss and sustain your interest in being fit. Don't just opt for the obvious ones, when you may find a totally new and surprising interest that suits you. There's nothing lost in going along to a trampoline session to find out if you like it, there are a lot more peculiar activities than bouncing your way to health; drinking yourself to death is one of them, it's just more conventionally peculiar.

OPTIONS

I haven't talked about team games or water sports or boating for beginners or hang gliding or riding or a whole host of things you might get excited about as you get fitter. The point is, as is the point with everything in this book, to use your imagination and think for yourself about what your body might be particularly good at or what you might like to try even as a one off. The principle is to get some exercise first so that you can benefit and develop your sporting skills. I believe in women getting involved in any activity that allows them to meet other women outside of the home focus, for the same reasons that I would prefer it if exercising women joined gyms or clubs; we get confidence from one another.

USEFUL CONTACTS AND BOOKS YOU MIGHT ENJOY

WALKING
    The Ramblers Association,
1–51 Wandsworth Rd, London SW8 2LJ.
The Race Walking Association,
Bridge Farm, Halstead Rd, Stanway, Colchester, Essex.
The Long Distance Walkers' Association,
29 Appledown Close, Alresford, Hants.

Books
    Walkers Britain, Pan, £4.95.
Walkers Handbook (H. D. Westacott), Penguin, £2.50.

RUNNING
    Women's Cross Country and Road Running Associations,
10 Anderton Close, Bury, Lancs.
Women's Amateur Athletics Association,
Francis House, Francis St, London SW1.

Books
    Running (Liz Sloan and Ann Kramer), Pandora Press, £4.50.
Running Magazine, 57–61 Mortimer St, London W1 (on sale last Thursday in the month).

SWIMMING
    Your best bet is to contact the Women's Amateur Athletics Association (see above) or to get in touch with your local pool or Sports Centre and find out what's on offer. Swimming books aren't that much use if you need stroke correction or lessons in the first place.

CYCLING
    Cyclists Touring Club,
Cotterell House, 69 Medrow, Godalming, Surrey.
National Bike Club,
c/o British Cycling Federation, 16 Upper Woburn Place, London WC1H HQE.
Bike Events,
PO Box 75, Bath, Avon.

SQUASH   Women's Squash Racket Association,
                    345 Upper Richmond Road West, Sheen, London,
                    SW14 8QN (SAE required).

MARTIAL ARTS   The Martial Arts Commission,
                    1st Floor, Broadway House, 15–16 Deptford Way,
                    London, SE8 4PE.
                    British Tai Chi Association,
                    7 Upper Woburn, London, W1.

SKIING   The Ski Club of Great Britain,
                    118 Eaton Sq., London, Sw1W 9AF.

MISCELLANEOUS   *Outrageous Acts and Everyday Rebellions* (Gloria
                    Steinem).

CHAPTER 5

BEHIND THE SCENES

We are all in the gutter, but some of us are looking at the stars.

Oscar Wilde

Now that you are fully confident about exercising and eating your way into the future; now that you've ordered your brand new bike and Speedo swimsuit, taken up hill walking at weekends and booked your cross country skiing holiday, you might like to know how to take care of your body in private, when it's just you and a toilet bag and a list of extras on offer at your gym. The work you put in behind the scenes will give you a fair share of the limelight because you'll look and feel well groomed and comfortably cared for all of the time. It's a bit more of the indulgence side that's so important in your preservation of yourself. True, your body can age, it's ageing from the moment you're born, but if you work with it, you can waylay the ravages of time before they waylay you. That doesn't involve hiding yourself behind a mask of make-up, just as your new body no longer needs a wardrobe of carefully chosen clothes before it appears the way you want it to be, you can strip yourself down to basics and take extra care of your most precious asset:

SKIN

Skin is often the first thing anyone notices about you, so you need to keep it as clean and healthy as possible. The best way to achieve this is to thoroughly cleanse it twice a day; when you get up in the morning, and last thing at night. If you live in a grimy city you'll be advised to use a deep-pore cleanser as well as soap and water. The cleanser will dig down into the pores and help to clear out bits of pollution and grime – the sort of problems that make skin look dull and lifeless. After you've wiped over with the cleanser (don't forget your neck), wash vigorously with a soap that suits your skin type – any old soap might well have a drying effect that you'll have to spend extra time combating with moisturizer. Your body itself, while not needing the same total cleansing process as your more exposed face and neck, will benefit from a rub down with a bath-mitt. Exfoliation removes the top layer of dead skin from the body leaving behind fresh glowing cells. Once you've passed thirty the time it takes for new cells to work their way to the surface of the skin is already taking around 25 per cent longer to happen than it did when you were in your twenties, so if you suffer from skin problems as you get older, they're going to be evident for that much longer unless you help the body out by exfoliating regularly. A facial scrub is obviously a good idea for the face, but there's no reason why you shouldn't use it on the rest of your body once a week, particularly if you have greasy skin that tends to hoard dirt; exercise always helps your skin to renew itself because sweat acts as an exfoliator. When you have your shower after working out, a rub down with a bath mitt or even a salted flannel will ensure a healthy cleaned out skin, that will go on looking younger for longer. Sluggish circulation that comes about with little or no exercise is always reflected in the skin, so you can be sure that while your workout is toning up your body shape it's also toning up your skin. Whilst skin is waterproof and apparently quite tough, it is extremely sensitive to excess of diet (spots) and nicotine (wrinkles). Women in particular need to be more careful about skin because our hormonal levels affect the amount of water the skin can carry – which it needs to stop it drying out – and our supply of collagen (supportive fat tissues that help give our skin its shape). Once collagen is thinned or weakened you can't replace it naturally and its loss is one of the disadvantages that beset serious dieters. Lack of it produces sagginess and hollowness around the eyes, in younger women a sure sign of insufficient nutrition. The other factor that skin really loathes is stress. The kind of psychological stress that women undergo in the modern world is anathama to our bodies. They rebel; and that rebellion apart from headaches and lethargy and chronic bad temper with physical side effects, shows itself in the skin. Dry skin gets drier and oily skin gets oilier. Rashes, dry or weeping, eczema, a slower ability to heal up cuts and minor wounds are all stress signs and obviously you should look for the source of that stress as well as trying to alleviate the problem for your skin. If you are under stress, you need more than ever to eat properly and to exercise, these two simple processes help the body to regulate itself which from your point of view will mean sleep and greater energy. If you know that your skin breaks out in any way when you're stressed, keep it as clean as you can, soaking it in water before you apply any creams, antiseptic or moisturizing. Your skin has to have water to hydrate, and remember that because your body is at least 50 per cent water, you should be drinking plenty of it. Skin likes six to eight glasses a day! Taken straight, and preferably mineral water of some kind. If your skin is oily, change your pillowcase often, and don't, no matter how wretched you feel, put your hands over your face. Your hands are nearly always full of dirt and bacteria and your facial skin will soak these up.

Women are fanatical about skin, spending huge amounts of money on any and every product that offers to lessen lines, clear blemishes and apparently improve the body's surface. Some of them may help, and certainly you should invest in good quality cleansers and moisturizers, with an occasional face pack to pep you up. Face packs have no real long-term effect, but they do temporarily improve the circulation and tighten the cells leaving you with a healthy glow. Skin reflects the way you live, and if you live badly, your skin will show it. Too much booze and salt both cause puffiness, especially under the eyes that eventually turns into permanent bags. Too much strain and too many late nights bring on the extra lines, and if you're in the habit of not taking your make-up off, you're setting yourself up for blotches and inflamed blood vessels. There are a variety of arguments about sunbeds and sunshine which I'll touch on later, but it seems to me that living well is more important to skin vitality than worrying about being in the sun.

WHAT YOU NEED

For the face: plenty of soap and water twice a day, followed by a moisturizer that suits your skin. When you wash, wash vigorously and if you live in a grubby town, use washing grains or a scrub or a deep cleanser. Steam clean your face once or twice a week. It's boring, but it's the cheapest and most effective way of ridding your pores of unwanted dirt. Don't do this though if you have acne or broken veins. It only serves to spread the infection.

There's no need to spend money on face masks when yoghurt, plain and straight out of the fridge will do just as well. It's soothing for sunburn or inflamed skin and it doesn't leave you with that constricted feeling as the face mask dries. Keep it on for around ten minutes and wash off with warm water. If you've got some cucumber in your fridge, cut a couple of slices and lay them over your eyes. Potato is just as good, especially for puffiness, but you might not like the smell. While you're lying down covered in yoghurt and cucumber try and clear your mind of all stressful thoughts, indeed any thoughts at all, except for pleasant day dreams. The mind needs to relax and it can't always do this when you sleep, so a bit of conscious slowing down will do wonders for your equilibrium as well as your skin. If strawberries are in season, eat them. You don't need to look at or concentrate on strawberries, which is fortunate, since your eyes are cucumbered, but they are the most wonderful thing for relaxing the body. Eat them slowly giving your homespun face mask and eye reviver time to work well.

Be sensitive to the weather. Skin responds to conditions outdoors and may need more attention if it's very cold or very sunny. Watch your skin carefully, it's the best meter you have of how your body's coping both with what you're putting into it and what you're asking from it. Well cared for, well fed skin will adapt easily to most weather conditions that are natural to it. If you're going abroad, give it some help because our skins are designed for where we live not where we holiday.

For the body: if you're exercising regularly, your body will respond well, keep the blood circulating and your skin shining. Help by exfoliating thoroughly with salt or a good soap. Apparently, soap isn't used very much by people who prefer baths to showers. They sit and soak, rather than wash. Your body needs washing, but if you've started exercising you'll be taking more showers than baths, which are better for your skin tone, and more likely to induce you to actually get clean. Remember that swimming in particular, because of the chlorine, dries out the skin, but any vigorous exercise requires that you replace some of the moisture you've sweated out. Buy a rich massage lotion of some kind and apply it liberally every time you work out. You'll find a rapid improvement in skin texture and softness. Spend extra time rubbing it into the backs of knees, elbows and bum – sensitive spots that chafe and dry out easily. One of the best things you can give your skin is a fresh or salt water swim and, failing that, the odd cold shower will tighten your pores and boost the blood supply to the surface cells. You'll emerge literally tingling and once you've got over the initial shock, you'll feel great.

Living well involves thinking about your body. If you notice how your skin reacts under certain conditions you can help it to overcome those conditions. Inflamed, hot feeling skin can often be the result of acute dehydration and irritation due to too much booze over a sustained period. So you stop altogether until your skin recovers. If you have a cold or an ailment that makes your skin feel sore to touch, give it plenty of soothing lotion and treat it extra gently – at such times it's a good idea to lay off coffee or tea and drink only mineral water. To purify your blood and therefore enhance and heal your skin, use a herbal remedy like dandelion root, or find a herbalist who will make up a tonic for you. This may seem a bit drastic, but if you've let yourself get out of condition on the surface as well as underneath you need to clear yourself out and start again.

For the hands: hands need hand cream. Hands get wet, dirty, dried out, toughened over and subjected to every kind of experience, so they deserve to be treated well. You don't have to spend a lot of money on hand cream, just make sure you're not allergic to whatever you choose. Money isn't always the deciding factor anyway, many cheaper brands are just as good as the ones with the flashy labels that cost three times as much. Experiment. Hands need cleaning too. Most people think that because they wash the rest of themselves and their clothes and the car and the dog with their hands, that their hands must be clean. Not so. If you look carefully, particularly if your hands have a large number of lines, you'll see how dirt can build up and lodge in the creases. The best way to give your hands a proper cleanse is to scrub them with a soft nail brush, well soaped. If your hands are discoloured, use a squirt of lemon juice or even a pumice stone. When you've done this rather drastic process, make sure you put on plenty of cream and then don't do anything for about fifteen minutes that involves your hands. This is amazingly difficult, but cunningly quite good for you because it means you'll have to sit down and relax.

To care for your nails, you should first be careful where you put them. Too much hot water, especially with harsh detergents, weakens the tough surface of the nail, causing splitting and cracking, so wear rubber gloves if you're doing prolonged or arduous handwork, and give hands a thorough cleanse when you've finished. If you do suffer from fragile nails nail varnish can help to protect them from chipping on a daily basis, but it won't solve the problem. You need a nail conditioner and plenty of Vit. A in your diet. So increase your stocks of carrots, eggs and cod liver oil. The cuticle – the skin at the base of the nail is very important because it determines how the nail grows. Push the skin back gently with a cotton bud to keep away from the nail itself and don't miss it out when you put handcream on the rest. Never poke the cuticle with a file and never use a metal file on the nails at all.

Your nails, like your skin, reflect your lifestyle. Anything that alters the natural balance of the body will show up on the surface areas. Stress not only leads to dull skin, it leads to nail blemishes and discolouring. Nails that are too soft or too brittle usually have their causes in diet. Too little zinc, calcium, B6 or iron will all affect the nails to their detriment, so make sure you're getting an adequate supply of leafy greens and low fat dairy products. If you have just come off the pill, or if you are going through the menopause, it's a good idea to supplement your diet with a Brewers Yeast tablet every day. Hormonal changes badly affect the condition of the nails, but you can assist the body in rebalancing itself by eating thoughtfully, keeping clear of irritants (alcohol and cigarettes) and getting plenty of rest. If your body is readjusting it can do without dashing around at the same time.

THE TROUBLE WITH FEET . . .

The trouble with feet is that they weren't intended to live inside shoes. Sweat builds up and stays trapped which helps bacteria to breed. This is smelly enough in itself but it can also lead to unpleasant rashes and athlete's foot. Socks or stockings need changing every day and you should rotate your shoes so that you don't wear the same pair two days running. Obviously, leather shoes with leather insides are much better for you than any synthetic material, but you should make sure that shoes are comfortable. Feet hate being squashed or bunched up, and if you must wear heels compensate your feet by taking them off (the shoes, that is) whenever you get a chance and at the end of the day, soak your feet in hot water. If you're the sort of person who tends to be on your feet a lot during the day, and goes straight out from work in the evening, it's a good idea to take a pair of shoes with you to change into, preferably ones that support your feet. If you sprain your ankle, slap an ice pack on it as quickly as possible and put the injured member on a stool for at least a day. If you try to hobble around you'll only make it worse. Chemists and health shops now sell general purpose foot lotions which cool, sooth and banish lurking bits of yuk from between the toes. If you want to keep your feet in the best of conditions, and doing exercise does demand more care, get one of those ointments and use it often. Most of them have some kind of herb content which revitalizes tired feet and leaves you feeling much fresher. An all over weekly massage will tell more about your feet than any other method. Feet like being rubbed and you'll soon discover any lingering soreness or incipient blistering. Women's feet don't smell as much as men's, but they tend to be in poorer condition, probably because of the shoes we wear, which aren't designed for an active lifestyle. In your pursuit of the good things in life, you need healthy feet, so take a critical took at yours and if there are any serious problems, like ingrowing toenails or verrucas, visit a chiropodist

(Greek for Foot-cutter), then stock yourself up with new socks or tights, and promise your feet freedom at least at the weekend. Tired or swollen feet affect much more than themselves, they make you bad tempered and out of sorts. You can't expect to have all the energy and health you want if any part of you is showing signs of disrepair.

GETTING AHEAD

You may not think that hair needs much attention apart from a good wash and a style that suits you; yes and no to both. Washing hair isn't just about getting hair clean; when you wash it you stimulate the growth cells and massage the scalp, so it's vital that you choose a soft shampoo that won't cause you more harm than good. Cheap supermarket brands are often nothing more than abrasive cleansers that leave your hair bereft of essential oils and smelling distinctly artificial. If you exercise and need to shampoo your hair every day, you should buy a more expensive health shop type that's gentle on your scalp and acts as a partial conditioner. Even with these shampoos you must rinse thoroughly and add a full conditioner at least twice a week. Conditioners thicken and strengthen the hair, leave it shiny and manageable and are not optional if you care about the quality of your mop. As far as a cut goes, that's up to your individuality, but you might try something more adventurous in your new life, especially if you're used to having it permed or artificially set in some way. A natural style is easier to handle and you don't have to worry about it growing out, plus you won't find it so difficult to keep soft. Hair matters. Dull hair can't be disguised despite all efforts to colour and style it. If it's dull, it's dull and the only thing you can do is give it a thorough overhaul and inspect your diet to check whether or not you're getting enough essential vitamins and minerals. If you're hair does look truly awful, or if it tends to turn limp and lifeless every so often, try changing to a range of haircare products like the ones offered by The Bodyshop and use them regularly for a couple of weeks. During this time give yourself a total henna treatment, you don't have to use the coloured variety if you don't want to, but the henna powder itself is probably the best revitalizer you can get. It's like feeding drooping plants Baby Bio. Doing it properly takes time because you have to sit wrapped in hot towels, but while you're sitting there comfort yourself that the heat is stimulating your scalp as the henna works on reforming the hair. Supplement this treatment with lots of green veg. and wholegrain products, and if it's winter, try and keep your hair snugly under wraps when you brave the elements. Healthy hair can take most changes of climate and temperature, lifeless hair just gets worse.

CHAPTER 6

THE BRAN TUB
Sex and a series of ideas to dip into . . .

He tells you when you're wearing too much lipstick,
And helps you with your girdle when your hips stick!
Ogden Nash

SEX

Sex is good for you and physical fitness makes you a better giver and taker of pleasure because your senses are heightened. There's no doubt that living actively enhances your ability to appreciate the world sensually, not just bodies, but everything you can touch and feel. Warm water, hot stone, summer rain all become pleasure sources in their own right and you'll probably find that as you get fitter you'll become more physical. You'll want to touch more, to use your body as well as your brain to quantify and experience. Animals and children use their bodies all the time to tell them about the world they're encountering, as we get older and literally more thick skinned we tend to ignore our body perceptions and go for the information received by the mind. Our five senses which should be directly linked to body awareness can become nothing more than channels for the brain and if this happens we're obviously missing out on a lot of enjoyment. If you want better sex you should consider the whole pleasure spectrum, including other people's bodies but not exclusively so. Start to handle things consciously, feeling their textures and weight, notice your own response to different things, how much pleasure do you get from stroking an animal or picking up a rare book? The attitude you have to your own body will obviously affect how much pleasure you can give and take from someone else's. As your body becomes the way you want it, you will desire yourself and have confidence in your powers as a lover. If you know you're beautiful other people are going to find you so. Many women complain of embarrassment about their figures, that their tummies are too large or that their breasts are too droopy. Such attitudes aren't going to make for relaxed and fulfilling sex and they're certainly not going to make for exciting sex because you'll feel you have to do it in a particular position with the light out. When you start to work out, you're starting a process that is sensual by its very nature. It may not feel that way at first, but soon you'll start enjoying moving your body, enjoying it develop and you'll want others to appreciate it with you. That's why it's so important to wear clothes you feel sexy and powerful in when you train. You're designing a new you and that new you amongst other things will be infinitely more attractive because your first priority is to become more attractive to yourself. That's body confidence and it's the best confidence you can have. When it comes to meeting potential lovers, you may have suffered from shyness in the past because you felt that your body wasn't up to romantic scrutiny; being fit, you can forget abut that and concentrate on whoever you're with knowing that if it does lead to sex, you're going to have a good time.

Exercise is aphrodisiac. Whenever I work out I want to make love because my body feels taut and alert and very happy, so expect an increase in desire when you take up fitness and possibly orgasm on the job. Women come very easily during exercise, and quite invisibly, so you may find more personal pleasure than you bargained for. Of course, if you have a lethargic lover who can't cope with your increased libido and general healthy physical responses, you may have to have an affair, and that may affect your life rather dramatically, but you didn't expect to remain the same after all your effort anyway did you? If you don't want to take another lover and you do want more sex, there's always masturbation which is a relieving and relaxing stand by. Masturbation is good for you even if you're getting enough sex from your partner because it reminds you how desirable you are and it teaches you all kinds of things about your body responses and what your body really enjoys. If you aren't fit and you feel very out of touch with yourself, you'd do well to include masturbation in your general fitness programme – not in the gym, obviously, but at home when you're giving yourself time alone.

The quality of your sex life improves beyond measure as you develop your muscles and increase your stamina. Crudely, you can do it for longer which is always a pleasure and if your pelvic muscles are tight and strong you'll feel everything on the inside much more powerfully. To maintain muscle tone in your pelvic floor, contract your buttocks as often as you can, it doesn't show and you'll be doing yourself and your partner a favour. As far as positioning goes, there are as many variations as you can manage and what might have struck you as absurd a few months ago will prove comfortable and erotic to your new fit self. Sex can become dull most easily when it always feels the same, when you can't vary the intensity or your response. Living well sexually involves pushing yourself to strange heights of pleasure and danger, experiencing sex in ways that use more muscles and more imagination. Forget the sex manuals, you don't need someone else's diagrams to show you how to enjoy your body, let your body tell you what it likes; you will learn to trust it via getting fit, it will no longer be an unreliable alien that you cover in as many clothes as possible. Your body can't embarrass you sexually and you shouldn't give a damn about telling your lover what feels good to you, especially since a whole variety of previously unthought of things are going to feel good. You may find you like to make love in the shower or upside down or straight after your evening run when you're still glowing and sweaty. You may find that you get so randy in the gym that you have to get a taxi home in order to save some innocent instructor from the full force of your lust. It's possible that you'll have a sexual revolution and want it all the time wherever you are. It can be done out of doors if you're careful. All that's happening is that your body's saying YIPEE, you've set it free at last and like the genie in the bottle, there's no going back.

A DAY OF REST

Give yourself a holiday, just for one day and preferably a week day so that you'll feel really pampered. Do any shopping the day before, so that you've got all the food you need, including some treats. Tell everyone you'll be away and take the phone off the hook just in case. The night before, go to bed early and forget about the alarm clock. Wake up in your own time, and when you wake remember that you don't have to leap out of bed, you only have to get up and make a cup of tea and go right back to snooze a bit more or read a book. When you finally decide to emerge have a shower and cover your body in all the things you like best, so that you feel and smell great. Put on your favourite comfortable clothes and make yourself, very slowly, the kind of breakfast you usually reserve for fantasies. If you want champagne in your orange juice, put it there. After breakfast, go out for a walk, preferably somewhere green and for as long as you like. If you want to fall asleep in the sun, do that, and if it's pouring with rain or windy, don't worry, just enjoy it anyway – it doesn't matter today if you get wet. Try and have lunch out, somewhere you feel comfortable in by yourself, and somewhere you can eat good food. Then the afternoon's up to you; cinema, a swim, more of that book, letters you'd been meaning to write to far away friends. Let your imagination run away with you, so that whatever you decide to do with the time, it's what you want. If you feel like eating a piece of cheesecake by mid-afternoon eat one.

When evening comes, you might like to do some gardening, or re-pot a few plants or hang a picture you've had lying around. You might even enjoy cleaning your bicycle. Do something almost active that gives you a sense of pleasure, then you can watch TV, steam clean your face or just pour yourself another glass of wine before you decide what to eat with your mange tout. Sweet dreams.

BREAKFAST TIPS

Women are the worst breakfast skippers, perhaps because they diet more than men and so believe that eating less is good for them. Breakfast is vital, it gives your body the fuel it needs to start the day and get moving again after anything up to twelve hours in bed. If you don't eat in the morning your blood sugar will fall rapidly and you'll soon be on the nibble. You might protest that eating anything at the ungodly hour you have to get up makes you feel sick, but if you can eat breakfast on holiday, or in a relaxed situation, what you're really objecting to are your early morning conditions, not the meal. You don't have to eat masses and you don't have to cook anything. Here are a few options:

1   Yoghurt with fresh fruit and honey. If you don't like yoghurt try the Greek variety which isn't low fat, but tastes wonderful. This combination will give you energy and plenty of vitamins and if you can add a slice of wholemeal toast, you've got your carbohydrate too.

2   If toast and a sweet spread is all you can manage, make sure the bread is wholemeal and go for honey rather than processed jams. Don't cover the toast in butter. An apple or banana on the way to work will help.

3   Boiled eggs, scrambled eggs or poached eggs on

toast are a good once or twice a week breakfast; you don't want to get egg bound.

4 Beans on toast, especially if you buy the wholefood variety of beans which sounds silly, but they taste better than anything else and they're good for you. This breakfast will give you plenty of fibre and protein and should be eaten in times of stress and followed by an orange.

Actual packaged breakfast cereals aren't much use and tend to be high on calories (including muesli), because they're loaded with sugar, so be a bit more imaginative and read the packet before you buy.

If you really have to run out of the house one morning and you know you won't be able to eat properly, at least grab a piece of fruit and some bread and stuff them in your pocket. Otherwise the chocolate biscuit urge might just become too much. Danish pastries are no better. What your drink with your breakfast is up to you, but you'd do your body good if you gave it a glass of mineral water on rising and before you throw down the tea or coffee. That sluggish almost sick feeling that belongs with mornings can be alleviated by a simple glass of water, it's all your body needs to allow it to detoxify and rehydrate your system. When you feel happy, at a weekend or on a day off, don't ruin it for your body by deciding to have a fried breakfast. Sausage, egg, bacon and fried bread can add up to nearly 1000 calories in themselves, which is a hefty amount unless you're about to go cross-country skiing. The cholesterol content is also too great for your body to handle, you're literally swamping your system in fat. If you want to know what your innards look like after that lot, drop a piece of kitchen roll into the pan and watch it soak up the fat. That's what you're asking your body to do. If you feel sick, you deserve it.

Treat your body well in the morning and you'll have a surprisingly easier day, even your usual irritants will seem less impossible and that's because you're properly fuelled, properly watered and properly cleaned out. Plus, if you've decided to make time for a real breakfast, you've been able to sit down and give yourself time to wake up, something that's very important after sleep, when the body and all its functions have been only ticking over. That extra half hour that you don't spend on your bed of pain, feeling like death, will give you more energy first thing than you've managed to achieve by midday. It's an investment, and it pays off.

TO SUN OR NOT TO SUN

What a question, and opinions are still as heated as the sunshine you're supposed to be staying away from. Doctors argue about skin types that need total block, skin types that should live in a portable tent, whether or not sunbathing brings on premature ageing, whether or not it causes skin cancer. There are a whole host of relatively untested questions with rather unsatisfactory answers. I would advise you to use your common-sense, your own awareness of your body and bear in mind one or two points before you bare your body.

High intensity radiation does cause the skin to age but you can prevent serious damage by building up your suntan slowly and making sure your skin is properly protected. Just because you don't burn doesn't mean you're not drying out. There are a whole host of reasons to seek the sun and it would be a pity to spoil any of the benefits by being careless.

In the days before antiseptic creams, sunlight was used to clear up skin ailments and eruptions, because ultra violet light reduces the amount of bacteria present in the skin which means that infection can't spread; this is why acne sufferers often report a clearing of even very bad patches when they find themselves in strong sunlight for a sustained period. Sunlight supplies you with Vitamin C which is vital for bones and teeth, and appears to affect the quality of the hair, though we don't know how. So if you want your hair to grow thicker quickly, take it to the sunshine. So much is said about the problems associated with sunshine that we don't spend enough time realizing how much good it does; it keeps us cheerful, which has the side effect of lowering stress and blood pressure, and it makes us randier which can only be a good thing since sex, too, lowers our habitual stress factor and promotes first rate circulation to all parts of the body. Make sure you have the correct protection factor suntan lotion and a good after sun moisturizer and never try and sunbathe with sunburn. You'll blister horribly and it's hard to live well covered in blisters.

MYTHS AND LEGENDS

CELLULITE

This doesn't exist, what does exist is too much fat that isn't properly supported. Getting rid of the fat and shaping the muscle underneath should remove the problem, including the crinkly effect that comes with it. So don't waste your cash on cellulite creams, nothing is going to take it away except hard work and sensible living.

THE PILL

The pill can cause water retention, so you should be especially careful over the amounts of salt and sugar you consume, both of which intensify the problem. The pill troubles the metabolism but exercise will help it to adjust and deal with any fluid retention or undue heaviness. Personally I think you should use the cap and forget all that romantic rubbish about spontaneity. How spontaneous do you feel with a water-logged body?

PERIODS

Exercise won't do anything to relieve stomach cramps unless you can relax a little to start with. If your body is ultra tense it won't respond well to exercise. The best stretchers for you to try are the leg-ins detailed on p. 25. Do them very slowly and if they don't work retire to bed with a hot water bottle.

113

FASTING   Forget it.

SUGAR v.   Honey is still sugar and if you start to put it into
HONEY   your tea instead of sugar you haven't cut your intake
                   at all, you've just altered the source.

SUNBEDS   You'll find almost more opinions about sunbeds
                   than you will about sunshine. They don't give you a
                   protective tan, that's for sure, but whether they're
                   especially bad for you is debatable. There are now a
                   number of products that claim to stop any drying
                   effect on your skin while you use the bed. I've tried
                   them out and they seem to work. My own feeling is
                   that I like to keep a tan once I've gone to all the
                   trouble of getting it and a weekly dose of sunbed
                   does just that. They're also great for your morale
                   during winter when all your colleagues are wander-
                   ing around looking like plague victims. If you're
                   desperate for the sunbed experience then go ahead;
                   you'll soon find out if it doesn't agree with you.
                   Remember you must wear goggles.

FOOTWORK   Just because you have the kind of job that requires
                   you to be on your feet all day doesn't mean you're
                   getting enough of or the right kind of exercise.
                   Certainly it's better for your body than sitting down
                   (sitting down doesn't much agree with bodies, they
                   prefer to lie or be in motion), but you still need to
                   take the weight off your feet and exercise the rest of
                   you.

PREGNANCY   You will benefit from exercise until very late on in
                   your pregnancy, though you should get special
                   advice as you get bigger about what would be good
                   and less good. This is where gyms and clubs, rather
                   than home workouts, are so useful. You'll have
                   trained help and you can ask your instructor to
                   design a programme around both your pregnancy
                   and your current level of fitness.

BACK UP

Your back has 50 bones, 100 joints, 1000 muscles and ligaments and over 100,000 nerve fibres. It supports the head, rib cage and limbs, and still manages to stay flexible. When you stand up, the whole of the upper part of the body is balanced on the lumbo-sacral joint – a joint about 3″ square. Not surprisingly, then, the back is extremely sensitive as well as extremely resilient to strains and pressures – it's very easy to injure your back, just by being careless, and if you do that, no amount of residual fitness or glowing skin is going to help. So along with your manic cycling and determined exfoliating, consider your back before your back lets you down.

If you stand badly you maximize the risk of back injury. Drooping shoulders force the neck to arch backwards instead of allowing it to balance easily and centrally. This arching will give you plenty of shoulder ache and neck tension and can help you to slip a disk if you stand badly and move suddenly. The other big standing sin, very common amongst women is pelvic tilt, that's where the tummy sticks out one side and the bum protrudes out the other, this puts a lot of strain on your 3″ joint, so pull in the tummy, straighten the shoulders and hold yourself upright. If you have an acute posture problem, you'd be advised to take up Tai Chi or the Graham Technique, both of which will slowly realign you and teach you how to use your back properly, at rest or in motion. If you just occasionally feel yourself standing sloppily, try and correct it as it happens and concentrate on your posture during exercise. You must employ parallel lines in order to lift weights and to do most floor exercises safely, so if this is a tricky area, take extra care, otherwise you could find yourself with a slipped disk instead of a brand new body.

Whenever you lift anything, particularly if your back is on the long side crouch down to it, and hold it close to your chest before you stand up. If you stoop, you're much more likely to pull a muscle. Suitcases and briefcases are terrible things because they concentrate the load unevenly, forcing your back to twist out of alignment. If possible, distribute your load so that the body carries it evenly. This can be difficult if you're in an office situation where two briefcases would look rather odd, but in all other situations, shopping or holidays or shifting equipment, go for two bags rather than one, and if possible use a rucksack which will evenly distribute your load.

If you often get aches and pains in your back, try swimming regularly. Removing the force of gravity from your body generally and your back particularly will allow the muscles to expand and relax. Yoga is another good method if you prefer something a bit more contemplative and if you want to go all out to strengthen your back, perhaps because you have a dream to trek across the Himalayas, then the form of Karate known as *Shotokan* which is based on a series of powerful kicks extending from the bottom of the spine, is exactly what you need. When you choose your personal exercise programme, you must take into account the state of your back and give it what it needs both for reparation and development. If you have a history of back trouble, don't start weight-lifting until you've had it checked out by a doctor or osteopath. There's no doubt that exercise will alleviate most back problems, if you allow yourself enough time and pick the right method. If you feel any pain in your back during exercise, stop immediately, stand upright and breathe deeply. It may be that you have just trapped a muscle, but pain should never be ignored, it's a signal for help, and as far as your back's concerned, you can't be too careful.

YOU ARE WHAT YOU EAT WITH

Most of us are so relieved when compulsory visits to the dentist end with childhood, that we can hardly bring ourselves to go back unless something really goes wrong. This is a mistake because teeth need a check up every six months, even if they feel fine and look the appropriate white colour. If you have a calcium deficiency your dentist will spot it in your teeth before you do, and you'll have plenty of time to put it right. If you leave it until you notice it, you've probably got about a week before all your teeth fall out. That's an exaggeration, but I have to terrify you into making an appointment if you're a reluctant dentist goer. If you've got any bleeding of the gums you should go at once.

Toothpaste is not a supermarket matter. Ordinary advertised toothpastes contain sugar to apparently make them more palatable to our overblown western sweet tooth, but clearly, extra sugar is just what your teeth don't need. For a really effective totally good for you toothpaste, try one of the health shop brands, like 'Tom's Natural Toothpaste' or 'Blackmore's Herbal'. They cost about four times as much as the other stuff but that doesn't seem to me to be a lot to pay for ultra healthy teeth and gums – they smell better too. When it comes to choosing a toothbrush, you have a bewildering array vying for your cash. Don't choose a brush that is too large for your mouth or too hard for your gums, an Oral B or Sensodyne is probably safest and they come in lots of different sizes. If you clean your teeth twice a day, you should change your toothbrush every 3 months, otherwise the bristles lose their resilience and won't clean your teeth properly. It's quite useful to buy toothbrushes in bulk so that you can cater for yourself and any unexpected guests who forget. Sharing toothbrushes might seem romantic but it's not very hygenic.

I'm ambiguous about Dental Floss. I know that it's wonderful stuff but I can never bring myself to use it. This is my failing, so if you can manage it, do so, and I'm sure you'll feel a lot better. Mouthwashes are another mysterious region, but these I have a lot of time for, not because I'm convinced they actually do what they're supposed to do, but because they make me feel better. They're a mental stimulant that allows me to challenge the world defiantly because I feel wholly clean. The real answer to bad breath does not lie in a bottle, nor in a tube of toothpaste, however expensive, it lies in what you eat and drink, not counting garlic which has a very pervasive smell that we would find pleasurable if we were Europeans. If you eat healthily, and don't drink too much alcohol your breath will smell sweeter than if you gobble up take-aways washed down with neat scotch. Mints at the end of a meal out do help if you're hoping for a night of romance, and the truly desperate should always carry with them a pack of those minty mouth fresheners that chemists sell in handy handbag sizes. After a rich lunch, the best thing you can do is to clean your teeth, eat an apple and drink a glass of water. If it's garlic you must get rid of, then the only effective way I know, and I've tried a vast number ranging from lemons to potato skin (raw) is to place a handful of tea leaves in your mouth and move them around as best you can; I don't know that the sort of tea you use matters very much, but I do know it's a very unpleasant process and best avoided. After you've done it, you drink water in order to spit the tea leaves clear. Definitely not to be done in company and definitely not (unlike garlic) an aphrodisiac. Teeth like to chew and crunch. They work best and keep in prime condition on hard fruit and veg., preferably raw. Ryvita suits them too, and if you're a worrier, crunchy foods will help you release your tension as well as please your teeth and gums.

ARMPITS

What makes you smell and what can you do about it? When you sweat your body is interested in losing heat to keep you cool, it's not exuding nasty waste matter, that's done via the bowels. If your skin is full of debris, dead cells and bits of dirt you haven't managed to wash off, you will smell when you sweat, since sweat is literally lifting off dirt as it pours out of you. If you exercise regularly, you won't smell bad because your skin will be continually shedding its dead bits, so your pores will stay clean and open, and the sweat, which isn't unpleasantly scented in itself, will leave the body easily. Sweat itself does get to be unpleasant if you've eaten the kind of foods that have a lasting aroma. Onions or alcohol in quantities will produce their own odour via the bloodstream and this will be manifest when you sweat. Too much coffee can have the same effect.

Shaving your armpits helps because it minimizes the jungle-like area in which bacteria can flourish. A clean shaven armpit will allow the sweat to pass out freely, collecting nothing unpleasant on the way. If you do shave, be careful about applying deodorant straight after, your skin is now ultra sensitive and may break out in a rash if you don't give it time to settle down. If you have touchy skin anyway, an average deodorant may be too strong and you should try something like the Body Shop brand, which contains less artificial ingredients and works just as well. Naturally, it costs more.

As you become fitter, your sweat pattern will change. The fitter you are the more quickly you will sweat during strenuous activity, so that your body keeps cool. The composition of your sweat changes too; it dilutes so that you lose less mineral salts as you perspire, and perhaps most important of all from a cosmetic point of view, your body will always smell sweeter. After all, sweat is part of our scent attraction, so if you find you're getting more attention for no apparent reason, look to your armpits.

EMERGENCY REMEDIES

What do you do when you wake up one morning looking and feeling like death, even though you're not ill? If you've got puffy tissues you're water-logged, so get a skipping rope and skip, this may sound ridiculous but it forces the blood into the face, and the blood will help clear excess fluid. Then run to the sink and swill your face in warm water followed by a deep moisturizer. After that you'll want to sit down. If your eyes are bad, too, cover them with cucumber or potato. If you look pale and dead tired and you want to look glowing and vital, take a cold shower, jumping up and down to keep yourself warm. This will promote circulation and certainly help you to wake up. Follow it with a large glass of freshly squeezed juice mixed with mineral water. If you're still not convinced try vigorously massaging your face with your fingers to regain colour. If all else fails, head for the make-up. Spots are a bore, but they happen to the best of us; if you can refrain from fiddling with it you'll have a chance of getting rid of it quite quickly, providing you clean it and cover it in antiseptic cream. My own answer to a real, nasty spot that I'm no way going to be able to disguise is to make a feature of it; buy yourself a kit of brightly coloured plasters, the sort that make kids feel better when they fall over and choose a colour to match your outfit, then slap the plaster over your spot. Such defiance will make you feel better and although everyone's going to ask what you've done, once it's covered up you can lie as much as you like, say the parrot bit you, or that a piece of glass flew into your bedroom as you were looking for clean socks. No one will doubt your word, they won't dare, and probably by the end of the day it will have started to go down. They need attention do spots. . . . If your hair stands hopelessly on end, make that into a feature too – gel it and go to work with pride. The rule is if it can't be covered up, flaunt it.

BODY RUBBISH

There are a lot of gimmicks on the market to help you get fit because we live in a gimmicky society. One of the worst is the machine that offers to tone you up electrically while you lie back and think of England. I hate this machine because it totally negates the idea of well-being. Muscles are there to be used and enjoyed, not artificially cajoled into shape. The benefits of exercise are more than skin-deep; there's the whole chemical reaction and response set up by your body when you work out. Machines don't ask you to take responsibility for your diet and your movements, they claim that you can live as you like and they'll do the job for you. At least in this country we aren't quite into stomach stapling and intestine by-pass surgery – yet, but the machines and the diet pills are offering the same disturbing opt out attitude. The diet pills don't fuel your body, diet biscuits and processed diet food aren't fuel at all, they're junk. Machines that give you electric muscle massage are junk too. You might as well be a cow or a battery hen. Every time you choose what looks like a short cut, you're saying that your body isn't worth the effort, that you don't want to consider your lifestyle, that all you want are results, not the pleasure in the doing. Exercise and living well pivot round the pleasure in the doing. There are no wonder ways to live well, it's a conscious, daily choice and each day you do it ensures another day of being able to do it. It builds. Passivity in the face of anything is a problem, and whilst you may not be a machine worshipper or a pill and two biscuit woman, don't get sucked into the fitness package passive exercise programme either. Gyms and workout classes are wonderful and the basis for your revolution, but you need to get outdoors, on a real bicycle, in the river or sea, for a walk somewhere pleasant. These activities may not add much to your actual physical régime, but they'll do amazing things for your temperament and overall happiness. You're creating a body that can experience and appreciate more life, so give yourself more life.

BRAIN POWER

If anything goes on behind the scenes, it's brain work, but nothing else has quite such an impressive effect on how you organize your life and present yourself to the world. Assuming that you're making a decision to get fit, and thereby improve the quality of your life in all areas, you'll want to think closely about what you're doing and how best to channel all your resources into a single and successful whole. Just as you must devote time to your body as a primary consideration, i.e. exercising it for its own sake, not just moving it around to enable you to do various tasks, so you must devote time to your mind in a similar way and for the same ends. The mind is more than a problem-solving survival plant, it's a creative source for your pleasure and development. You don't have to join one of the numerous and growing contemplation or encounter groups, you don't have to meditate for hours, all you have to do is give your mind time to make its own connections.

Being alone with your mind can be quite a daunting process. You may be witty and intelligent, and well able to hold forth on any matter, you may be genuinely able to use other people's ideas to inform your own; the corrective of dialogue is very useful but it can't be fully useful if you don't leave time for yourself to think in new ways. When was the last time you went for a walk by yourself, not to work anything out, but for the sheer pleasure of your own company? When the mind is always subject to company or trauma, when it is only used as a social machine or a personal computer it grows slack. It does what you ask of it very well, but its other functions, which are rather more exhilarating, get left behind. Try taking a piece of paper and start to write on it before you have time to think what you might like to write. This may be slow or look stupid at first, but as you begin to cover the paper, you'll be able to watch your mind forming new wholes; finding links where there weren't any and showing you how much there is going on inside. The mind is a relentless synthesizer despite the fact we usually ask it to analyse – to take things apart so that we can look at them. If you allow it, your mind will take your world, break it into pieces around you and spin it in front of you in shapes and colours you hardly recognize. This need not be frightening; you still have your memory to tell how something used to look and you can always dismiss any disturbing connections as part of the game you are playing. In some ways it is a game, in so much as all of ordered reality is a game, a series of constructions we use to save ourselves from chaos. It's real, but it's also relative because it's the way we want things to appear to be at a certain time. Alter the time and you alter the perception (Quantum Physics argues that this formula is reversible, alter the perceptions and you alter the time. I haven't the scope to go into time travel here, but you might like to). You might be wondering what this has to do with your well-being; it has to do with it quite crucially because just as you understand how a limp body leads to a limp life, you should also understand how an underused brain spoils the many pleasures that might be yours. When you allow your mind to follow its own tracks, rather than the ones you set for it, your world can only become more imaginatively biased. Whatever you touch upon will gain extra relevance as your mind shows you by irresistible synthesis, how relevant to you most things can be. You can use almost anything to improve your life once you learn how to process it into your experience. Just as cacti detect water deep in the earth's crust, you will detect pleasure and relevance from the most unlikely sources. You will look about you and see the same things differently. Moments of vision are only that; seeing the same things differently. A heightened experience need not only belong to artists, it can belong to you in the same way that the sheer physical pleasure of your body belongs to you as you begin to develop it. You know that such things are no longer the preserve of athletes, and artists, after all, are mental athletes, they use their minds differently.

Of course, the correlate of pleasure is danger. It's dangerous to let your mind loose because you might not want the old ways of seeing, and that might mean altering your life, but you have already started to alter your life, every time you give priority to a body you used to ignore, you are altering your life. This is no small undertaking, but it is a chance to live well . . .

INDEX

PANDORA PRESS

**CHANGING
LIVES**

Our selection of Handbooks designed to represent the changing lives of women today is growing fast.

YOUR BODY, YOUR BABY, YOUR LIFE
by Angela Phillips
with Nicky Lean and Barbara Jacobs
From the co-editor of the English edition of OUR BODIES, OURSELVES, a non-patronizing, non-moralizing, non-sexist guide to pregnancy and childbirth.
0–86358–006–8 222pp A5 illustrated with diagrams and cartoons

RUNNING
The Women's Handbook
by Liz Sloan and Ann Kramer
With illustrations by Jo Nesbitt and Elaine Anderson
A handbook for the hundreds and thousands of women who run or want to start running – enabling women to lead a fitter, freer life.
0–86358–943–2 138pp illustrated

DISCOVERING WOMEN'S HISTORY
A Practical Manual
by Deirdre Beddoe
'An invaluable and fascinating guide to the raw material for anyone approaching this unexplored territory.' *Sunday Times*
0–86358–008–4 232pp illustrated

ON YOUR OWN
A Guide to Independent Living
by Jean Shapiro
A bible for all divorced and widowed women, covering all of the practical and emotional matters that women are likely to face when they find themselves suddenly 'on their own'.
0–86358–027–0c   250pp   illustrated
0–86358–045–9p

NATURAL HEALING IN GYNECOLOGY
by Rina Nissim, translated by Roxanne Claire
A handbook of natural remedies for women's use in the treatment of a whole range of disorders, from PMT to cystitis.
0–86358–063–7c   200pp
0–86358–069–6p